Endorsements for *Big Picture Medicine*

With *Big Picture Medicine*, Dr. Porter offers a steady, supportive voice in an increasingly confusing world of health advice. This book helps readers feel grounded, informed, and empowered as they take meaningful steps toward vitality and optimal well-being.

David Perlmutter, MD, FACN

Author, #1 *New York Times* bestseller,
Grain Brain and *Brain Defenders*

After losing my dad to early-onset Alzheimer's eight years ago, I became serious about my own health and longevity. Dr. Stuart Porter helped me cut through outdated medical dogma and the endless stream of health advice to focus on the principles that truly make a difference. This book brings that wisdom together and shows why balancing our spiritual, emotional, and physical well-being is foundational to real health and longevity.

Allen Bolen

Jiujitsu IBJJF three-time world champion
Professional bowhunter

True wellness starts with understanding what our bodies actually need. In *Big Picture Medicine*, Dr. Porter connects nutrition, lifestyle, and root-cause healing in a way that empowers readers to take ownership of their health and build lasting habits.

Karalynne Call

CEO and founder, Just Ingredients

As a four-time Olympian and World Cup champion in alpine skiing, my career depended on understanding how the body performs, heals, and adapts. The principles in *Big Picture Medicine* align closely with what I've learned through decades of high-performance sport and personal health exploration.

This book takes a powerful big-picture approach to health—connecting lifestyle, mindset, nutrition, and emerging therapies into a practical framework for optimizing human performance and longevity. I've lived many of these principles myself, and I believe this book offers valuable insight for anyone looking to take control of their health and unlock their full potential.

Steven Nyman

Four-time Olympian and three-time alpine skiing
World Cup champion

As someone who cares deeply about understanding the why behind health, I really appreciate Dr. Porter's approach. He breaks down complex ideas in a way that feels clear, practical, and actually applicable to everyday life. This book is thoughtful, empowering, and a great resource for anyone looking to take a more informed and proactive role in their health.

Demi Engemann

Secret Lives of Mormon Wives

BIG PICTURE MEDICINE

Optimizing Health and Wellness Through Functional Medicine and Peptide Integration

by

Dr. Stuart B. Porter, DO

MAISON VERO

Published by Maison Vero
1619 Providence Road South, Suite 220-254
Marvin, North Carolina 28173

Inquiries may be directed to: Maison Vero, 1619 Providence Road South, Suite 220-254, Marvin, NC 28173, or info@graymilleragency.com.

For information about special discounts for bulk purchases, please call (949) 333-4872 or email info@graymilleragency.com.

Maison Vero is a partner brand of The Gray + Miller Agency, a speaking, literary, and talent consortium.

For more information on the talent represented by The Gray + Miller Agency, or to bring any of our thought leaders to your organization or live event, please visit our website at graymilleragency.com

Cover Design: Kelly Thompson
Book Design: Elizabeth Young

Manufactured in the United States of America

Paperback 978-1-969508-42-4
E-book 978-1-969508--43.1
Hardcover 978-1-969508-41.7

Dedication

To my family—whose love, patience, and encouragement have been my foundation. To my patients—whose courage and resilience have been my greatest teachers. And to all who believe that medicine can be more than managing disease—that it can be restorative, personalized, and transformative. May this book serve as both inspiration and a guide on the path to optimal health and well-being.

Table of Contents

Introduction

How healthy do you want to be?

It sounds obvious, but most people never really ask themselves that. We might say we *want* to be healthy, but we rarely stop to define what that means—let alone imagine what it would take to get there.

It starts with desire.

That's step one in any transformation. Can you picture yourself being truly healthy—not just "getting by" or managing symptoms, but feeling strong, clear-minded, emotionally grounded, and spiritually connected? Whether you're an elite athlete or haven't exercised in years, the truth is the same: We can all optimize our health and vitality. Ultimately, you can decide if you want good, better, or best health.

But what does healthy mean to you? The "answer" has been the subject of many books and deliberated on lecture stages for years. For some, it's as basic as not being sick. For others, it's peak performance, mental clarity, spiritual connection, and strong relationships. "Health" can mean something different for every person, depending on where they are and what they value. Before we dive in further, ask yourself: What does health mean *to me?* And once you've defined that, then ask: Where am I now in relation to that vision?

Health is not merely the absence of disease. True health is the presence of vitality. It's the capacity to fully engage with life—to think clearly, move freely, love deeply, and serve others meaningfully. When our health improves—especially when our physical, emotional, and spiritual health align—our ability to contribute expands. Whether you're a parent, teacher, nurse, leader, or friend, optimized health amplifies your capacity. It's not selfish to pursue optimal health; in fact, it might be the most generous thing you can do. The healthier you are, the more you have to give. In other words: *Your health isn't just about you—it's who you become when you're at your best.*

This book is your roadmap to optimizing health to be your very best. It explores education, motivation, and transformation and shows you the *why* behind the changes I recommend—because once you understand the why, change becomes possible. Meaningful. Longer lasting. And *attainable*.

The chapters ahead will walk you through key systems that define foundational health—digestive, immune, nervous, and mitochondrial. These aren't abstract concepts; they're real, tangible systems you can learn to support and optimize. You'll realize that health isn't just about avoiding illness but living with energy, clarity, purpose, and joy, creating a lifestyle that enhances well-being and longevity. This works—I've demonstrably lived it, creating a fulfilling, exhilarating life.

How did I get here? I grew up in a big family with seven children—five boys and two girls. I was the third boy, stuck right in the middle, and like many middle children, I learned early how to navigate the world in ways that didn't always make sense to adults. But I had a pretty big roadblock that made navigating more challenging. I was saddled with undiagnosed dyslexia, including a significant stutter that shaped my nascent years, particularly my relationship with learning and with myself. Speaking or reading aloud in class, for example, inspired constant anxiety. I'd come up with a host of excuses to avoid it—pretending I'd lost my place in a book, dropping my pencil, whatever it took not to feel humiliated in front of my peers. Of course, I didn't know this at the time. I didn't fully understand I had dyslexia until I entered medical school.

I hadn't even realized I had atypical inner workings. My brain was likely inflamed from childhood, and the way I demonstrated that was with dyslexia and subsequent stuttering exacerbated by teasing from others. But there were gifts hidden inside those challenges. The late Robert Redford's late son James directed a 2012 documentary, *The Big Picture: Rethinking Dyslexia*, to this effect, dispelling myths and misconceptions about dyslexia through a story about a high school senior chasing his dream of attending a competitive college. It's a powerful film that also features a cast including David Boies,

Richard Branson, and Sheree Carter-Galvan, who share their own challenges with dyslexia.

Dyslexia forced me to think differently; it trained my brain to notice patterns, to zoom out and connect dots that others might miss. That's how I see health today—not through a narrow lens but as a broad, interconnected system we can all learn to understand and optimize. It allows me to have that "Big Picture" view of health optimization.

In my case, my challenges didn't change until much later when I started learning more about dyslexia's cause and nuances, notably the connection of chronic inflammatory response syndrome—and how to treat it. Along the way, that knowledge improved some of the foundational concepts that health practitioners teach and practice in functional medicine.

At the time, I was entrenched in triathlon competition, doing everything I possibly could to get an edge up on my competitors, including a very strict anti-inflammatory diet to help optimize health and mitochondrial function. I even shifted over to a healthy version of a ketogenic diet for about seven years to enhance mitochondrial function and climb higher in event placings.

But in doing all those things related to diet and inflammatory response, my brain started working better. A couple of years into my new lifestyle regimen, I noticed that I could read better, faster. Reading, neuroprocessing speed, and focus all began gradually improving.

In the years since, I have dedicated my career to helping patients optimize their health at a cellular level, focusing on hormonal balance, metabolic function, mitochondrial efficiency, and longevity. And I can thank my mother for it. I attribute a lot of what guided my direction to functional medicine to her. She was very independent and forward-thinking, studying anything and everything she could related to holistic health—from herbology and homeopathy to iridology and reflexology. Later, she conducted extensive research on diets, and her seven children were the guinea pigs for her experimentation. Seeing the value of what that brought to our family piqued my interest in a more natural approach to medicine. As a kid, our family physician was an osteopathic physician like I am today—philosophically, osteopathy is a bit more holistic, treating the whole person and facilitating the body to heal itself. Ultimately, I got the best of both worlds. I matriculated into osteopathic medical school and had an Army scholarship that opened the doors into whatever specialty I wanted to explore.

Long before settling in Utah in 1995, I was an avid alpine skier, especially in the powder, and really took to backcountry skiing. The level of fitness required for the latter is significant. You climb thousands and thousands of vertical feet, descend, and repeat. After doing that for a few years and realizing I needed something in the off-season to keep my fitness at a high level, I started cycling. I bought a plain-Jane recreational bike, went out on a couple rides with family and friends, and realized "I'm pretty good at this." *Hmm, maybe I should try competing.*

I did some races and then hired a cycling coach who happened to be a professional triathlete. He eventually convinced me I could compete at a high level in that sport as well, and I went after it, notching multiple high placings in Ironman competitions, qualifying for a handful of Ironman World Championship qualifications and subsequent world championship competitions. I was obviously quite focused (one might say addicted) on winning or at least discovering what my old body could achieve through optimizing health and mitochondrial function. At the end of the 2017 Ironman season, I was ranked (then in the fifty-five to fifty-nine age category) first in the U.S. and fourth in the world. For those in the know, my VO2 max at the age of sixty-two was at 62. Obviously some of that is genetic, but I firmly believe that a functional medicine approach to optimizing health, and specifically mitochondrial health, helped my body achieve that level of health and fitness.

That's my short story on discovering the tri life, but it was all for the purpose of cross-training to stay fit for backcountry skiing.

However, being competitive by nature, I very much got caught up in the competition piece. Coming full circle, I used those experiences as a platform for my practice.

Since my heady time at Brigham Young University, I've dedicated two decades and counting of nearly forty years practicing medicine to the front end of pioneering medical advancements that enhance vitality, physical performance, and aging. I live this lifestyle to the fullest extent, and if this is what I can do for my health, then I can help you do something similar to optimize yours. My goal is to empower you to take charge of your health through education and a broader understanding of both modern medicine and spiritual practices, using practical tools and insights grounded in functional medicine, to optimize health at any age.

This book is my opportunity to give back and share what I've learned throughout the years, culminating in my roles as medical director and founder of Integrative Medical Associates and Xage Medical Spa, and as medical director of Haven Wellness, a peptide-focused supplement company. You'll learn what has worked for patients in my practice, as well as for me personally. Through that experience, I'll outline a health and wellness program that is practical, results-driven, and rooted in functional medicine—focusing on gut, immune, neuroendocrine, and mitochondrial health, which play key roles in boosting energy, slowing aging, and optimizing overall vitality.

One of the problems in our society and in medical communities is the tendency to rabbit-hole into specific issues. With the internet at our fingertips, it's easy to get lost in the weeds. Many people, especially those suffering from chronic inflammatory conditions, need better guidance. They need someone who can pull them out of those weeds, tell them what matters most, help them better understand the "order of things," and show them how to prioritize their journey to optimal health. By focusing on the foundational elements, we can provide clear steps for optimizing health.

Ultimately, this is our opportunity to consider the "miraculous molecules" in therapeutic peptides that can take our health to the next level. As we'll discuss in Chapter Nine, peptides dispense an extraordinary element of vibrant health:

- **Optimizing cellular regeneration** for anti-aging benefits
- **Boosting energy levels** by improving mitochondrial function
- **Accelerating recovery** from injuries and inflammation
- **Enhancing cognitive function** and neuroplasticity
- **Regulating metabolism** for improved body composition

It's not just about lifespan but health span—years lived in optimal health and function. You can make the changes that improve your health, well-being, longevity, and joy in life by building awareness and putting these principles into daily practice.

You already have everything you need to get started. What you need now is a clear plan, a little direction, encouragement, and the belief that it's worth the effort.

PART ONE

Understanding the Problem

Before becoming familiar with the *How* of health optimization, we need to understand the *Why*. Part One lays the groundwork by taking a closer look at the modern health crisis—and why so many of us are struggling despite access to more medical resources than ever before. At the heart of this crisis lies a silent, chronic condition that is often overlooked in conventional medicine: inflammation. Specifically, chronic inflammation, which underlies a staggering number of health issues today, from autoimmune disease to anxiety, fatigue, weight gain, and the list goes on.

Chapter One opens with a deeply personal story—one that moves from childhood learning challenges to competitive endurance athletics—and uses it to frame a key truth: Optimal health doesn't happen by accident. It takes intention, education, and effort. We explore how toxic exposures, nutritional depletion, and an overburdened immune system have created a perfect storm that makes vibrant health harder to achieve. You'll be introduced to chronic inflammatory response syndrome (CIRS), which affects nearly 1 in 4 people, and learn why symptoms like fatigue, brain fog, and thyroid issues may be part of a bigger story.

Chapter Two unpacks what it really means to be healthy—not just free of disease, but functioning optimally in body, mind, and spirit. Too often, we settle for "getting by" rather than asking what our bodies and minds are truly capable of. You'll learn about the five foundational pillars of health: gut health, immune function, brain and nervous system health, mitochondrial function, and spiritual/emotional well-being. Together, we'll begin to see how these systems work in unison—and why healing one often requires addressing all.

Chapter Three brings attention to a dimension most health books neglect: the role of spirituality in true healing. While supplements and strategies are powerful, lasting transformation often comes when our actions are aligned with deeper purpose and faith. You'll see how spiritual beliefs can positively influence everything from immune resilience to emotional balance and how Christ-centered healing can guide us toward restoration in every aspect of life. Through scripture, science, and personal experience, we'll make the case for a holistic model of care—one that treats the whole person, not just isolated symptoms.

Taken together, this section challenges us to see health not as the absence of illness, but as the presence of vitality—the ability to live fully, serve others, and thrive in body, mind, and spirit. To attain optimal health, we need both offensive and defensive strategies to navigate the fractured world in which we live.

Let's ramp up our health to the highest level!

CHAPTER 1

Why Are We So Sick?

We are drowning in information, while starving for wisdom.

E.O. Wilson

Once upon a time, it was better than this.

In the past, long before we migrated to living and working inside buildings, health threats weren't quite as prevalent. But today we live in a fundamentally different environment than our ancestors—one where we are constantly bombarded with toxins that didn't exist then. Every day, human-manufactured toxins permeate the air we breathe, the food we eat, and, of course, the plastic containers we use and drink from. Our interiors, while providing shelter, trap these toxins and concentrate them in our living and working spaces.

Food, for example, represents an enormous part of this toxic exposure. The food industry spends billions marketing processed products specifically engineered, through deliberate food addiction science, to hijack your brain's reward pathways and keep you coming back for more. Unless you eat with intention—to include the natural instead of the artificial—every meal is laced with ingredients that can potentially do you harm.

Beyond food, we continually face challenges from contaminated water supplies (a frighteningly grave concern given dwindling water sources and rampant overuse), air pollution, exposure to medications (including antibiotics that end up in our food chain), and electromagnetic frequencies (EMFs), or "electro smog," cellular networks and electronic devices that emit frequencies our bodies never evolved to process, absorbing them rather than combating their effects. This invisible pollution affects our biological systems in ways we are only beginning to understand. These EMFs deserve special attention, as they increasingly challenge our mitochondria and overall cellular health.

Social media represents another modern health disruptor. Beyond a host of documented mental health impacts, social media platforms can promote visual images that create unrealistic health and beauty standards and distort our perception of what health—and life—should look like. The images themselves may not be real, but they can have very real consequences on our mental, emotional, and physical well-being.

That's the crux of the problem: Much of the global human population functions at a level that gets by day-to-day, but it is far from ideal and, in fact, steers us down a path of inexorable deterioration. Optimal health, however, rarely happens by accident; it requires a plan, education, and concerted effort. The principles in this book are your starting point for that plan, including:

- A genuine desire for change
- The ability to visualize your healthiest self
- Education about your unique health needs
- A sustainable, personalized plan to optimize health

And most of all, maintaining a consistent effort. And not just a New Year's resolution-type effort—I'm going to do this for a couple of weeks and magically cut sugar from my diet or get six-pack abs or eat more vegetables. Achieving true health is an ongoing process. The ultimate goal isn't eliminating symptoms but creating a foundation for lifelong wellness.

At the core of most chronic health conditions lies chronic inflammation. Unlike acute inflammation—your body's normal, healthy response to injury or infection—chronic inflammation persists when the inflammatory response fails to shut off properly. This ongoing inflammatory state becomes the driver behind most chronic health problems we see today—autoimmune diseases, cardiovascular disease, stroke, Alzheimer's, arthritis, chronic fatigue, fibromyalgia, even mood disorders, which most definitively carry an inflammatory component.

This is all tied back to immune system dysregulation. People don't know which way to turn or where to focus because they don't yet have a big-picture view. Our modern medical approach operates on naming specific diagnoses and then prescribing treatments for each labeled condition. That approach only treats symptoms, not the cause of chronic illness. By doing so, conventional approaches may provide temporary relief but seldom resolve the fundamental drivers of disease.

We need to understand and address chronic inflammatory response syndrome (CIRS) so that we can move upstream to tackle deeper causes. For example, someone diagnosed with Hashimoto's thyroiditis—where the immune system attacks the thyroid—is experiencing a downstream manifestation of an inflammatory process. The autoimmune attack is a sign of dysregulation, not the primary problem itself.

Consider that inflammation drives virtually every chronic condition you can name:

- Arthritis
- Autoimmune disorders
- Cardiovascular disease
- Chronic fatigue syndrome
- Cognitive decline and dementia
- Fibromyalgia
- Mental health and mood disorders
- Stroke

What connects these seemingly diverse conditions? They all stem from underlying inflammatory processes.

All humans carry variants in the HLA-DR family of genes. Certain combinations of those genes predispose many people to immune imbalance that then opens the door for chronic inflammation. These genes can be identified through specialized testing, providing insight into one's susceptibility. Having these genetic variants doesn't guarantee the development of inflammatory conditions, but it does significantly increase risk. Conversely, people without these genetic markers can still develop chronic inflammation through other pathways. The takeaway here is that while chronic inflammation is very common, we can diagnose and treat it successfully.

Understanding the Inflammatory Cascade

Chronic inflammatory response syndrome (CIRS) represents much more than localized tissue swelling. It's a systemic immune imbalance that triggers cascading effects throughout the body.

In individuals susceptible to CIRS, this immune dysregulation creates a domino effect. (*See Fig. 1.*) The body receives the inflammation signal first, and then, unsure of what to do, its immune system gets stuck in a loop. The brain and pituitary gland also become inflamed, further disrupting immune function. Since the gut and immune system are intimately connected, gut inflammation typically accompanies this process—though determining which came first is often difficult due to their bidirectional relationship.

As inflammation spreads, various symptoms emerge. Eventually, these symptom clusters receive specific diagnoses like lupus, rheumatoid arthritis, fibromyalgia, and the list goes on. However, the upstream cause remains the same: immune imbalance initiating inflammatory cascades.

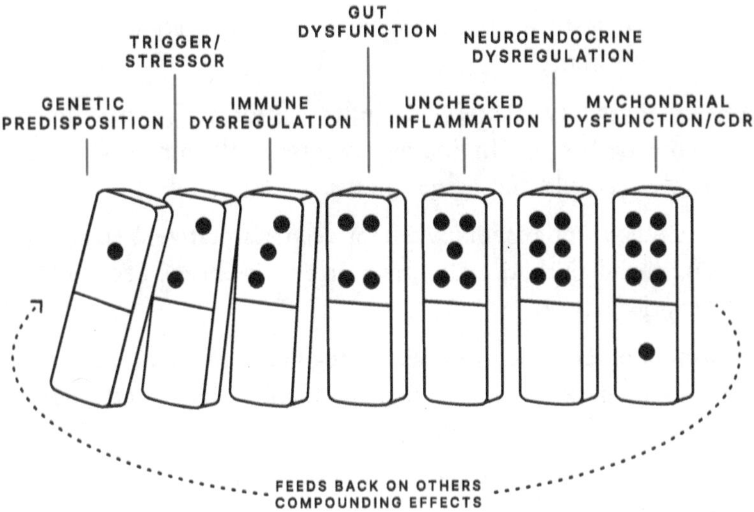

Figure 1. CIRS domino effect.

CIRS was initially called "mold toxin illness" when Dr. Ritchie Shoemaker first identified it in the late 1990s while studying patients who became ill after exposure to biotoxins in water-damaged buildings and algal blooms in the Chesapeake Bay area. He later developed what is known as the Shoemaker Protocol for treating CIRS,[1] and many practitioners still focus primarily on binding and removing these biotoxins. I commend Dr. Shoemaker for his brilliant discovery of CIRS.

However, newer approaches[2] focus on correcting the underlying immune imbalance rather than just eliminating toxins. By treating the dysregulated immune response with targeted interventions, including peptide therapy, we can address the root cause, yielding significantly higher success rates than by focusing primarily on biotoxin removal.

When we restore proper immune balance, the body regains its ability to recognize and process environmental toxins appropriately. This not only resolves current indicators but builds resilience against future exposures.

How do we do this? Addressing chronic inflammation requires a multifaceted strategy:

Anti-inflammatory Dietary Changes: Prioritize whole, nutrient-dense foods while eliminating processed, inflammatory triggers like sugar, seed oils, and refined grains.

Quality Sleep Optimization: Aim for deep, restorative sleep by supporting circadian rhythm, limiting screen time before bed, and addressing sleep disorders.

Appropriate Exercise: Engage in regular movement that supports lymphatic flow, reduces inflammation, and builds resilience—without overtraining.

Stress Management: Incorporate techniques like breathwork, meditation, time in nature, or therapy to reduce chronic stress, cortisol overload, and anxiety.

Targeted Supplementation: Use evidence-based nutrients (like omega-3s, vitamin D, magnesium, curcumin, and many more) to support immune regulation and reduce inflammatory pathways.

Advanced therapies like peptides, when indicated, leverage precision tools to modulate immune function, repair tissues, and support cellular communication when foundational strategies need additional support.

Hashimoto thyroiditis, a very common autoimmune illness, is an ideal example of what this looks like in real time. Most people diagnosed with hypothyroidism likely have Hashimoto's, though many remain unaware of it. That's because traditional medicine often bypasses testing for thyroid antibodies, focusing only on thyroid hormone levels. Practitioners check TSH, T4, and sometimes T3 levels, then prescribe replacement hormones without investigating why the thyroid is underperforming in the first place.

This approach misses the fundamental issue: Hashimoto's is an autoimmune disease where the body mistakenly attacks its own thyroid tissue—the very tissue responsible for producing hormones critical to metabolism, energy production, and countless other bodily functions. When we look upstream, however, we consistently find that these patients have genetic markers predisposing them to CIRS.

But through comprehensive blood testing, we can quantify the extent of inflammation, measure immune system imbalance, and assess inflammation in the digestive and respiratory tract linings. One particularly revealing marker I routinely check is the alpha melanocyte-stimulating hormone, a pituitary hormone that often serves as a barometer for broader neuroendocrine function. This is a big deal, as approximately 80 percent of my Hashimoto's patients, in my own practice, significantly underproduce this critical hormone, indicating deeper systemic dysregulation.

After establishing baseline measurements that confirm chronic inflammatory response syndrome, we can begin addressing root causes. First, we implement an anti-inflammatory diet tailored to the individual's specific triggers and sensitivities. This dietary intervention provides the foundation for healing by removing inflammatory inputs and supporting cellular repair mechanisms. Next, we optimize sleep patterns to ensure patients achieve truly restorative sleep. Quality sleep isn't merely a luxury—it's essential for mitochondrial recovery and immune system regulation.

In addition, the mental health component cannot be overlooked, as anxiety and depression frequently accompany inflammatory conditions. We address these aspects through stress management techniques, targeted nutraceuticals that support calm neurological function, and professional counseling when appropriate. This integrated approach recognizes that mental and physical health are inseparable aspects of the same system.

Then we get into foundational supplements, which play a crucial role, with omega-3 fatty acids from marine sources standing as perhaps the most critical intervention. I emphasize to patients that without adequate omega-3s, their other anti-inflammatory efforts will be severely compromised or fail altogether. Unless we consume cold water fatty fish multiple times a week, quality omega supplements must be taken consistently to effectively address inflammation at the cellular level.

Additional supportive supplements, including prebiotics and probiotics, help restore gut microbiome balance, which directly influences immune function and overall inflammatory status. This gut-focused approach recognizes the bidirectional relationship between digestive health and immune regulation, as well as the gut-brain connection.

By addressing these foundational factors rather than simply managing thyroid hormone levels, we often see improvement not only in thyroid function but across multiple body systems. Patients report increased energy, better mental clarity, improved mood, and reduced pain—benefits that extend far beyond what thyroid replacement alone could achieve.

Inflammation Manifested

When we talk about how inflammation affects the body, it's important to understand that the presentation varies dramatically between individuals, depending on which domino tracks decide to fall. This creates unique patterns based on genetic predispositions and individual vulnerabilities.

For some people, inflammation manifests primarily as anxiety—a condition that's often overlooked as a potential physical health issue. Others develop more recognized autoimmune/inflammatory conditions like Hashimoto's, typically experiencing associated fatigue and a general sense of "I just don't feel right" that impacts daily functioning. Many patients receive diagnoses like chronic fatigue syndrome or fibromyalgia, that, unfortunately, traditional physicians remain reluctant to diagnose or treat. It's a ubiquitous and systemic problem in modern medicine. First, functional medicine (root cause medicine) is not in mainstream medical school or residency curriculum. Our current system focuses on giving a diagnosis (label) to a particular set of symptoms and findings and then prescribing a particular pharmaceutical drug (or more than one) for that particular "diagnosis" rather than going further, thinking more broadly, and discovering the root/real upstream cause.

Unfortunately, the pharmaceutical industry has far too much influence on our medical school curriculum and our medical system at large.

Yet these conditions clearly stem from chronic inflammation and respond appropriately to anti-inflammatory and immune-modulating interventions.

The prevalence of these inflammatory conditions cannot be overstated. If approximately 24 percent of the population carries genetic predispositions to inflammatory disorders, and most of these individuals develop systemic inflammatory conditions, it's not surprising that roughly 80 percent of patients in my practice have CIRS. This represents most of the chronic conditions we treat daily.

The good news is that we can objectively measure this inflammation, precisely identify treatment targets, and implement comprehensive protocols that address the root causes. I typically follow up with patients every three to four months after initiating treatment and consistently hear encouraging reports of increased energy levels, enhanced mental focus and clarity, improved restorative sleep, improvement in digestion, reduced pain (joint pain, muscle pain, headaches, and migraines), and decreased allergic responses. We also consistently see demonstrable improvements in the immune and inflammatory biomarkers that we monitor.

These widespread improvements occur because we're addressing the fundamental immune imbalance that leaves the door open for inflammation. By successfully restoring proper immune function, reducing systemic inflammation, and restoring mitochondrial health, we create conditions for healing across multiple body systems simultaneously. This approach explains why treating inflammation at its source yields such comprehensive benefits—we are addressing the upstream drivers of numerous, seemingly unrelated conditions.

The myopic symptom-focused approach often leads to pharmaceutical interventions that merely mask rather than resolve. This prescription-first, "pill for every ill" approach has become so ingrained in our medical system that we rarely question it.

The proliferation of biologic drugs for autoimmune diseases perfectly illustrates this problem. Almost every month, Big Pharma peddles new medications to physicians, who then prescribe them to patients as a silver bullet for their ailments. The drugs also appear in direct-to-consumer television advertisements, promising relief for specific inflammatory conditions. While these medications effectively reduce discomfort, they merely blunt the immune system.

Ultimately, this approach generates billions in revenue for Big Pharma for managing—but never resolving—chronic conditions, without advocating any real lifestyle change or even generating improvement in health. Yes, symptoms might improve (although they are predominantly only masked), but at what cost?

Consider someone suffering from active ulcerative colitis who begins taking biologic immune suppressants. The medication quiets the acute inflammation, providing welcome relief, but simultaneously increases vulnerability to infections and boosts cancer risk as these medications compromise the immune system.

The very system designed to protect us becomes compromised. That's just not good medicine (or least not good comprehensive holistic medicine).

By contrast, maintaining a comprehensive perspective that focuses on root causes helps identify upstream factors that drive inflammation—whether dietary triggers, sleep disruption, environmental toxins, stress, or gut dysbiosis. Addressing these foundational issues, from "how do we reduce a patient's inflammation" to "why is this person inflamed in the first place," not only improves current conditions but also prevents future manifestations of the same underlying problem.

The difference lies in physicians' willingness to step back and investigate why the body is responding with inflammation in the first place. This approach requires more time, broader thinking, and patient education, but it ultimately creates genuine healing.

True healthcare must evolve beyond our current fragmented paradigm toward a model that prioritizes addressing root causes—creating sustainable wellness rather than merely suppressing the body's signals that something deeper requires attention.

Most people settle for feeling "fine"—but fine isn't the same as thriving. In the next chapter, we'll explore the crucial difference between simply avoiding disease and truly achieving optimal health—because there's a whole other level of vitality waiting when you stop chasing normal.

CHAPTER 2

Health vs. *Optimal* Health

Medicine should not just add years to life but add life to years.

George Engel

Consider this revealing example from my practice. A seventeen-year-old patient, Lysa, came to me struggling with two years of chronic pain most everywhere in her body. She'd been seen by a pediatrician and had been found to have a low white blood cell count. A positive anti-nuclear antibody test raised suspicion for autoimmune disease, suggesting the immune system was producing antibodies against the body's own tissues. Additional reported symptoms included:

- Debilitating fatigue
- Anxiety, depression, and OCD tendencies
- Chills, sweats
- Dizziness, near-fainting
- Brain fog and concentration difficulties
- Insomnia and poor-quality sleep
- Unintentional weight loss
- Migratory numbness and tingling
- Bloating, diarrhea, and reflux

The pediatrician thought that the rest of Lysa's labs were "normal" and diagnosed her with amplified musculoskeletal pain syndrome, another term for fibromyalgia. However, after just six months of switching to our treatment protocols that incorporated an anti-inflammatory diet, emotional and spiritual healing, sleep optimization, and peptide therapies, Lysa dramatically improved to become more social, expressive, and positive, with a desire to guide others toward optimal health. Since then, hers has become an oft-referenced example of root-cause, systems-based healing, now embodying what it means to experience optimal health—physically, emotionally, mentally, and spiritually.

What distinguished this patient journey wasn't her age but her extraordinary commitment to transformation. Unlike many adults who approach health improvements with hesitation, she embraced our protocols completely—including a rigorous anti-inflammatory nutritional approach that would challenge most grown individuals. This approach went far beyond simple compliance; it reflected a deep conviction that healing was possible. Within just four months, her transformation was remarkable—energy surged, mental clarity sharpened, emotional balance stabilized, sleep deepened, and digestive symptoms resolved. And these weren't just subjective improvements—her follow-up bloodwork confirmed significant shifts in her biological markers.

The key difference? She possessed a clear vision of possibility. She wanted more than just symptom relief; she sought a comprehensive vitality.

In our modern world, we have fragmented the once naturally integrated, powerful relationship between mind, body, and spirit. We've advanced technologically at breakneck speed, and continue to do so, but simultaneously disconnected from the holistic understanding of wellness that guided human health for thousands of years. This separation has profound consequences on our well-being that we're only beginning to recognize.

What does it mean to be "healthy" versus having truly optimized health? Although the answer can be independent to someone's vision of optimal health and lifestyle, most people today settle for a baseline level of functioning—getting through their days with just enough energy and clarity to meet their responsibilities. This standard of "healthy enough" falls dramatically short of our inherent potential. True optimization doesn't happen by chance; it emerges from intention, understanding, and persistent action.

True optimization doesn't happen by chance; it emerges from intention, understanding, and persistent action.

Lysa's story illustrates the fundamental distinction between conventional "health" and true "optimization." For some people, being healthy could be "I ate a banana today and walked around the block, so I feel great," and often means avoiding diagnosable conditions. Optimization manifests as reaching your fullest potential across *all* dimensions of being. Your mental state affects your physical body, your physical condition influences your spiritual awareness, and your spiritual well-being shapes your mental outlook—an intricate relationship where no element exists in isolation.

The pathway to optimization is a matter of where you want to take it and includes:

- Developing a compelling vision for your life health
- Trusting the process of transformation
- Gaining personalized insights about your unique needs
- Creating sustainable practices that honor your individual constitution

Remember that your journey toward optimal health isn't about quick fixes or generic protocols. It begins with fundamental questions: What future do you envision for yourself? What quality of life do you desire? What potential do you wish to fulfill? We can provide guidance and frameworks, but commitment and vision determine whether you'll move from adequate to better to best.

The mind-body-spirit connection is the concrete foundation upon which extraordinary health is built. Understanding and honoring this relationship is your second step toward thriving, every day.

You've already taken the first step by picking up this book. You feel there's more to health than simply avoiding disease, you understand that the journey requires commitment, and you're prepared for the challenging work ahead. You are here because you want to make changes and have an idea of what that might mean.

We have a unique practice here. Most of our patients find us by word of mouth, referred by friends, colleagues, or family members, and they have a strong appreciation of what we're going to outline for them and the level of commitment it will take to see results. The difference in comparison to traditional medical practice is that the majority of our patients are already committed, and because of that, our compliance and success rates are quite high.

Whatever your choice of a sport or hobby or goal—triathlons, cycling, backpacking, gardening—you do it at a level you want to achieve. The distinction between conventional health and true optimization mirrors the difference between casual participation and serious commitment in any pursuit. Whether someone takes up cycling for weekend rides or trains for a competitive race depends entirely on their vision and dedication. The same principle applies to health—you can maintain basic function, or you can pursue extraordinary vitality.

But there's a catch. The mental and emotional components of this journey often prove the most challenging territory to navigate. These aspects require deep introspection into where limiting beliefs originate, how they impact various areas of life, and what fundamental shifts in identity are necessary for lasting change. When you're ready to identify who you want to be, and align your actions accordingly, you can do what you need to get there. In the process, you not only learn new things about yourself and your inner strength but also how it manifests into that end result of where you want to be, which can impact your daily life, habits, fulfillment, and even the people around you. It's a lot of work, but if you put shoulder to the wheel and commit, you'll get there.

Transformative Change Starts Here

Keep in mind that it often takes a significant challenge—a health crisis, personal setback, or moment of reckoning—to ignite the necessary fire for change. These trials can humble us enough to listen, motivate us to seek new approaches, and provide the spiritual catalyst needed for genuine transformation. The hope is that difficulties become triggers for positive change rather than reasons for surrender. Some people fold under pressure, losing faith in their capacity for improvement. Others discover that challenges reveal their true potential. The difference lies not in the severity of the obstacle but in the response it generates—whether it diminishes hope or strengthens resolve.

The pathway to optimization requires full engagement across all mind, body, and spirit dimensions. Integration is essential, as physical protocols without mental commitment produce limited results. A spiritual mindset without practical application remains incomplete. Mental focus without physical foundation lacks sustainability.

This begs a fundamental question: Are you ready to move beyond the desire for change to fully embody it?

The first step starts with physical health, the foundation for overall well-being. We'll identify the physical symptoms that often indicate deeper emotional or spiritual imbalances, positioning the body as a critical component of healing. For example, there's a condition known as cell danger response (CDR),[3] which is associated with chronic inflammation and mitochondrial dysfunction. From a broad, big-picture perspective, the cell danger response is triggered when the body experiences significant stress that can be physical, chemical, microbial, or, as is often the case, emotional in nature. Trauma, in particular, frequently serves as a catalyst for this response.

While an inflammatory challenge alone—such as exposure to environmental biotoxins like mold—can activate the CDR, in my experience and studies, it's often an emotional or psychological trigger that initiates the cascade. This aligns with what we discussed in the first chapter about immune dysregulation and getting "stuck" in a chronic inflammatory state.

CDR is a real, biological mechanism; it's the body's innate cellular response to perceived environmental threats or injuries. It shifts cellular metabolism in an effort to protect the cell and the organism as a whole. While adaptive in the short term, if CDR is not resolved, the body can become trapped in a maladaptive state of inflammation and dysfunction.

Healing from this state often requires more than addressing physical symptoms; it requires healing the trauma that initiated it. This can happen through various modalities: counseling, somatic therapy, spiritual practices, biofeedback, and, in some cases, medical interventions. In our clinical setting, for example, we sometimes work with individuals who have significant PTSD or unresolved trauma by offering IV ketamine treatments. Ketamine, a dissociative anesthetic with psychedelic properties, facilitates a kind of neurochemical reset, promoting neuro-regeneration to help rewire maladaptive patterns in the brain. This kind of reset is often key to helping the body shift out of the cell danger response.

We can design the most detailed and disciplined healing protocols, but without addressing the emotional and spiritual roots of the issue, true and lasting healing often remains elusive. This is why we emphasize a multifactorial, multifaceted approach. You have to look at it from every angle—physically, emotionally, spiritually.

When we help the body reset from the CDR—what you might think of as a neuroendocrine, emotional, or spiritual reset—the body can begin to heal. And real healing is only possible when we recognize that the body is a partner in a deeply integrated, whole-person journey toward well-being.

Foundational Health

The latest and greatest directives for establishing a bedrock of enduring health are ubiquitous in the nutritional healthcare space. I've built a four-part foundational structure inspired by the Word of Wisdom, a conical scripture from section 89 of the Doctrine and Covenants from the Church of Jesus Christ of Latter-Day Saints. These God-given health recommendations, which I've nicknamed Heaven's Health Code, include what to abstain from and what to frame within our diet, "to be used with prudence and thanksgiving," outlining the critical importance of gratitude.

In essence, the God-given food pyramid (*see Fig.2*) presumes the order of the listed food groups from the bottom of the pyramid to the top. "Every herb in the season thereof, and every fruit in the season thereof" emphasizes the importance of a variety of produce. "Yea, flesh also of beasts and of the fowls of the air, I, the Lord, have ordained for the use of man with thanksgiving: nevertheless, they are to be used sparingly." And last, (top of the pyramid), "All grain is ordained for the use of man and of beasts."

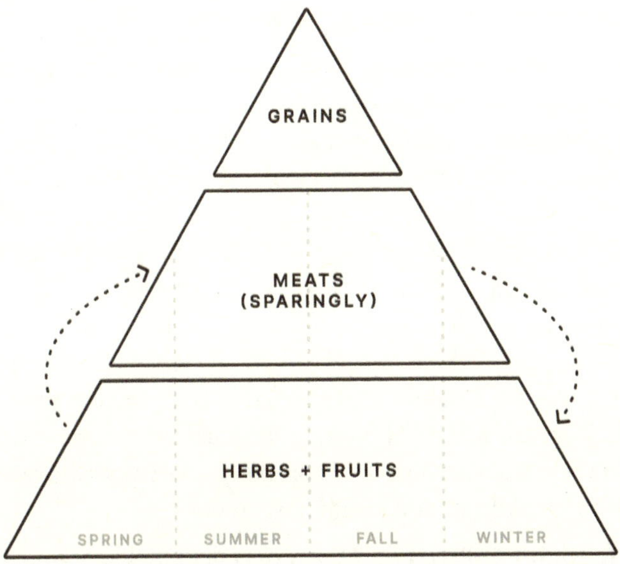

Figure 2. God-given food pyramid.

After the food pyramid is a list of associated blessings for those who obey/comply with the four-part structure mentioned previously—"shall receive health in their navel, marrow to their bones, and shall find wisdom and great treasures of knowledge, even hidden treasures, and shall run and not be weary and shall walk and not faint." (This last blessing correlates with mitochondrial health, and I believe it is an invitation to exercise regularly to further optimize health.) Translated to whole health, the code shapes out like this:

- Gut health (health in the navel)
- Immune health (marrow to their bones)
- Brain-central nervous system (wisdom and great treasures of knowledge)
- Mitochondrial function (run and not be weary, and walk and not faint)

Fascinatingly, this is how a functional medicine approach actually works. Presuming that Christ is the author of this God-given health code, one might surmise that Christ, the Master Healer, knows "a little something" about healing and optimizing health!

While considering this God-given health code, let us remember that our bodies are truly sacred. As souls, bodies, and spirits, we are walking, talking, breathing, living, and loving miracles. Our bodies are the temples of our spirits. We are created in the image of God, supported by numerous biblical scriptures on the topic. Here is just one as an example: 1 Corinthians 3:16-17: "Know ye not that ye are the temple of God, and that the Spirit of God dwelleth in you? If any man defile the temple of God, him shall God destroy; for the temple of God is holy, which temple ye are." It's quite clear in just this one scripture that our bodies are sacred and we need to treat them as such. If we consistently keep this concept in mind, we should be more likely to nourish ourselves optimally—nutritionally, spiritually, and emotionally as God would have us do.

I will detail this in Part Two, but to start, let's look at foundational health, which I liken to a "health house," if you will, with each level representing a crucial element of well-being. Just as with a stable, lasting structure, whole health must have a solid foundation, but our goal is to be further optimized, making sure things are in order, then build to optimal. This model's blueprint includes four components: foundation, framework, interior, and roof.

Foundation (Core Health Behaviors)

Your health depends on a solid base of:

- Quality sleep
- Nutritious, balanced eating
- Regular physical activity
- Stress regulation
- Emotional stability
- Healthy relationships
- Safety and basic resources (shelter, clean water, financial security)

Of course, if the foundation cracks, everything above it becomes unstable.

Framework (Body Systems and Habits)

This is the structure of the framework, or "house":

- Cardiovascular health
- Immune system
- Musculoskeletal system
- Gut health and metabolism
- Brain and nervous system function
- Daily routines and lifestyle habits

This framework distributes energy and resilience throughout the body and mind.

Interior (Personal Goals and Preferences)

What makes your "house" feel like a home is:

- Joy, fulfillment, and hobbies
- Career or life purpose
- Creativity, spiritual well-being

- Interpersonal relationships/love
- Physical well-being/appearance or performance goals

This is where individuality and lifestyle expression shine—but they depend on the stability of the house's structure.

Roof (Protective and Advanced Measures)

The roof keeps outside threats from damaging your health:

- Preventive care (preventive exams/baseline testing)
- Supplementation/medications when appropriate and treatments
- Medical interventions or surgeries when necessary
- Access to care

The roof is important—but it's only effective if what's underneath is already strong.

As you can see, a holistic structure emphasizes interdependence—everything must be aligned and maintained. Clear priorities follow suit. You don't build a roof before a foundation. Likewise, you shouldn't chase performance or appearance goals before addressing sleep or mental health. Everyone's "ideal health" looks different, and this model respects personal choice—customizable interiors—once the basics are in place.

In similar fashion, the CIRS foundational recommendations I share with patients include an anti-inflammatory/sometimes autoimmune-type diet (foundation), stress management, restorative sleep (framework), omega-3s, brain support/regeneration, immunomodulation, gut healing (interior), and mitochondrial enhancement (the roof).

Directly related to these metrics, and a threat to generate cracks in their support, is the impact of stress and trauma on body and spirit.

When looking through a holistic lens, we can see the well-being of the whole person—body, mind, and spirit—guided by the ultimate healer, Jesus Christ. Holistic healing encourages practices that promote balance, such as nutrition, movement, emotional awareness, and mindfulness. These tools are incredibly valuable in helping us live more intentional, healthier lives. At the same time, there's a deeper kind of healing that involves our sense of purpose, connection, and inner peace. From a Christian perspective, this deep healing is centered on the life and teachings of Jesus Christ, who offered comfort, perspective, and renewal to those who were struggling—not just physically, but emotionally and spiritually as well.

When we bring the idea of Christ-centered healing into our wellness journey, it shifts our focus. Instead of pursuing health solely for personal gain or self-optimization, we begin to see it as a way to strengthen ourselves so we can better contribute to the lives of others. Taking care of ourselves becomes less about control and more about stewardship—preparing to be more present, compassionate, and generous. Whether it's through acts of service, encouraging someone in their own growth, or simply sharing what brings us joy and purpose, healing becomes a way to give, not just something to get. In this light, both holistic and faith-informed approaches can work together and enrich one another.

Ultimately, what motivates us at our core? Hopefully, it's not selfish ambition. I'll admit—at one point, my drive was just to win, win, win, no matter the cost. But over time, I've come to believe that real purpose comes from looking outward, not inward.

Instead of chasing success for its own sake, we can choose to be driven by a desire to contribute—whether that's serving others, uplifting those around us, or helping people achieve better health and well-being. That kind of motivation comes from a place of spiritual, emotional, and personal maturity. It's less about personal gain and more about making a meaningful impact.

Ironically, to serve others, we often have to focus on our own well-being first. Achieving optimal health—physically, emotionally, spiritually—does take some self-focus. But the end goal isn't just self-improvement. It's about being in a strong position to give more, to serve more, and to show up for others in a meaningful way.

For example, one of my sons started improving his own health, took up running, and began participating in marathons. That led him to join a running club, and now he leads the group—motivating others, organizing events, and encouraging them to experience the benefits he's found through fitness and community. It's been really inspiring to watch.

Another son has done something similar with backcountry skiing/splitboarding. After being trained and certified in backcountry avalanche safety, he started inviting people along to share the experience: the beauty of nature, the joy of movement, the love of health and fitness. It's simple but powerful.

Of course, service can take many forms. It might look like community involvement, church service, volunteering, or just encouraging someone to make a positive change in their life. The important thing is that our drive—our purpose—evolves into something bigger than ourselves. It comes full circle too; hopefully we'll have the desire and vision to improve our overall holistic health to better serve others. In doing so, we experience what I call spiritual momentum (which includes physical in this respect), as looking outward to serve, we are strengthened from within.

Best of all, helping others is a proven conduit to reducing stress, improving heart health, and even boosting immune function. For example, studies have shown that people (men in particular) who have had heart attacks are more likely to experience depression. But when that depression is addressed and treated, it helps to reduce future cardiovascular risk.[4] As we serve others, we are more likely to be emotionally healthy, and that normalizes cortisol levels, which positively influences our health and ability to recover.[5] We can look to the autonomic nervous system as well, the sympathetic and parasympathetic sides, which correlate to yin (sympathetic or fight and flight) and yang (parasympathetic or rest and restore) in Chinese Eastern medicine. Serving others stimulates the parasympathetic (yang) side of the autonomic nervous system with a restorative boost, something we need much more of in our modern world, where it's easy to have too much of the sympathetic fight and flight side and not enough parasympathetic.

In the same vein as service, gratitude brings another significant health impact, including social well-being, improved sleep quality, lower risk of depression, cardiovascular health, and even longer life.[6] While gratitude-related longevity is still being studied, recent research points to a lower risk of myriad physical and mental health-related causes.[7] It's no surprise that gratitude generally brings happiness, but it can also inspire greater focus on achieving and maintaining quality health. One effective method I practice regularly is that of regular daily prayer. I try to spend more time thanking God than I do in requesting blessings from Him. Additionally, I try to recommend to my patients to simply slow down and appreciate everything around them. Walking through a forest, hiking up a mountain, or just watching your kids chase butterflies all bring an infusion of goodness that makes a difference. I believe that God and His goodness are everywhere. We just need to learn to see it and appreciate it. Even in the trials we face, we can and should see that, in some sense, God may allow them in order for us to grow from those trials and adversities. Consider it as spiritual hormesis. It is through these trials that we see positive changes in our character. In that sense, we should be grateful for our trials.

Bringing it all together is the spiritual aspect of healing and wellness, which provides a sense of deeper meaning and motivation that can sustain long-term change. When individuals connect their health journey to a greater purpose—aligning with personal values, nurturing relationships, or feeling connected to something beyond themselves—they're more likely to stay committed to it. Understanding that wellness is not just physical, but also emotional and spiritual, helps create a more holistic and fulfilling approach. It turns health practices from routine checkboxes into meaningful acts of self-respect and stewardship, often leading to greater consistency, resilience, and overall well-being.

CHAPTER 3

Spirituality's Role in Healing and Health

A joyful heart is good medicine,
but a broken spirit dries up the bones.

Proverbs 17:22

At first, I just wanted to win. And I did "all the right stuff" with diet, supplements, and precise training to make it happen. Like in Chattanooga, Tennessee, 2017—arguably my best Ironman competition, and one of those rare days where everything just clicked. That's far from typical in an Ironman; you can almost always count on something going sideways. The distance alone—140.6 miles—guarantees that. Even in this race, there was still that inevitable dark point. No matter how fit or prepared you are, there comes a moment in a long, grueling race where you start to doubt yourself. *Can I really keep going? Can I push through this?*

But leading up to that moment, this event had gone unusually well. I'm not the strongest swimmer, and the swim is usually something I just try to survive. But in Chattanooga, the swim is downstream on the Tennessee River, and that made all the difference. It was fast. An inner tube thrown in the water likely would've moved as quickly as I did—but I was *moving.* When I got out of the water and checked my watch, the time was much faster than my usual. That gave me a huge jolt of confidence and set the tone for the rest of the day.

The bike leg felt smooth and strong, even in the classic Southern summer weather: thick humidity that clings to you like dried egg yolk on a breakfast plate and hot, steamy air that can't quite make it all the way into your lungs. It didn't matter; I was locked in and rolled into transition off the bike in first place. Exciting, to be sure, but it also comes with pressure. Could I keep it up? From there, it became a mental game: dig deep, stay steady, don't let adrenaline push you too hard too early on the run.

About three-quarters through the marathon, I hit that wall—the dark place. My legs were heavy, my mind was tired, and internal doubt whispered *What if I can't hold this lead?* Oddly, I dodged the doubt and instead felt a moment of joy. Not because anything got easier—my body was still hurting—but because I had a sense of *being in it*, fully present. There's something deeply human about testing your limits and realizing you still have more to give.

In that moment, I remembered a simple trick I'd picked up over the years: *force a smile*. Even if it feels fake, do it. So I did. And somehow, that physical act sparked something deeper that became palpably spiritual. The heaviness lifted, my stride smoothed out, I felt calm and energized. I knew I could finish strong.

I crossed the finish line 26 minutes ahead of second place, completely spent—but completely fulfilled. Preparation, mindset, and conditions all aligned that day. You don't forget a feeling like that.

On the other end of the spectrum, you don't forget the difficult times either. I'm currently serving as an ecclesiastical leader in a local LDS church. One of the things I've been learning through this experience is the real need to develop patience. In our faith, we're taught to pray for charity, meaning the attributes of Christ. However, praying for those kinds of attributes often opens the door to experiences that are anything but easy. In fact, they are usually quite difficult—and they're meant to shape us.

To wit: My wife and I took a trip to Mexico over a Christmas-New Year's season, and, unfortunately, I came back with a classic case of Montezuma's revenge—traveler's diarrhea. After we got home, I was impatient to heal, and rather than wait until the next day to get a safer, more familiar antibiotic, I decided to take a single dose of Cipro (short for Ciprofloxacin). It's FDA-approved for treating traveler's diarrhea, but I didn't fully trust it. Cipro is in a class of antibiotics known for an array of significant side effects, including, for example, the risk of tendon ruptures in the Achilles, rotator cuffs, and biceps. Personally, I don't even like seeing them on the market, but I was impatient and figured just one dose while waiting for the other medication couldn't hurt.

That decision sent my health into a tailspin. I lost twenty-two pounds in seventeen days and rapidly became dangerously undernourished. I had started with about 6 to 8 percent body fat, so I had no reserves—my body survived purely off muscle. I had taken Tums right before the antibiotic, only to later find out that this particular antibiotic doesn't absorb into the bloodstream when calcium and/or magnesium are consumed simultaneously. Instead, it concentrates in the gut lumen up to tenfold the usual concentration.

Ciprofloxacin is part of a class of antibiotics that, in some people, causes severe adverse effects, such as damaging mitochondrial function, and can even affect our DNA adversely. In my case, it caused something called bile acid malabsorption syndrome and completely destroyed the villi—those tiny hair-like projections in the small intestine. All the healthy flora in my gut had been wiped out and ushered in a firsthand experience of what it's like to lose the immune protection and stability that a healthy gut provides. I had lost my "health in the navel." It was brutally difficult and took months to even begin recovering. I'm still not back to where I was—maybe 90 percent there. The compromised gut health weakened my immune system. I ended up getting shingles, and it didn't stop there. The virus spread to my liver, causing hepatitis. The liver began to fibrose, inspiring a real fear that I might need to go on a liver transplant list. I was terrified.

I tried every medical and holistic treatment available—fecal transplants, peptides, you name it. Spiritually, it was incredibly humbling. I leaned heavily on God, priesthood blessings from family and friends, and on faith in miracles.

When we ask for things like patience or charity, we often don't realize what we're inviting. There's really only one way to gain those attributes: through deep, refining hardship. That's a good thing. I learned so much from and was grateful for this experience that will have an enduring impact on the rest of my life. By practicing patience and following my gut (pun intended), I saw the cascading effects of a single choice.

Holistic Meets Spiritual

At its base level, holistic healing is the interconnectedness of mind, body, and spirit. But is there a deeper meaning in the pursuit of optimal health? I believe there is, and it is found in alignment of the three. Examining how functional medicine aligns with spiritual practices cuts to the heart of everything we think we know about healing. For too long, we've compartmentalized our approach to wellness, treating symptoms in isolation while ignoring the profound connection between our physical, mental, and spiritual selves and their direct influence on one another. What if the missing piece in your health puzzle isn't another supplement or treatment protocol, but a fundamental shift in how you understand healing itself?

Holistic healing is the interconnectedness of mind, body, and spirit found in alignment of the three.

Patients who achieve extraordinary results refuse to accept "normal" as good enough. They don't just want their blood pressure to be acceptable or their energy levels to be adequate. They want their bodies to feel like allies rather than obstacles, with minds clear and spirits soaring. This vision drives everything else. When you're committed to extraordinary health, you make different choices about food, movement, relationships, and spiritual practices.

Understanding true healing requires us to examine the three interconnected dimensions that work together like components of nature's ecosystems. A disruption in one throws off the balance of the whole, but when they all thrive, we are blessed with vibrance and resilience.

The Emotional Dimension (Mind)

This is where most people get stuck, and honestly, where most healthcare providers feel least equipped to help. The emotional dimension of healing requires you to examine not just what you feel, but why you feel it, where those patterns originated, and how they're serving or sabotaging your health.

Your emotions aren't just psychological experiences; they are events that create measurable changes in your body chemistry. For example, chronic anger floods your system with inflammatory chemicals; persistent fear suppresses immune function; unresolved grief can literally break your heart, manifesting as cardiovascular disease.

But the paradox is that the emotions that seem most destructive often carry the most important information. Your anxiety might be pointing toward something in your life that needs attention. Your sadness might be honoring a loss that deserves to be grieved. Your anger might be protecting boundaries that need to be established.

Healing happens not when you eliminate these emotions, but when you learn to work with them skillfully. This requires courage because it often means facing parts of yourself you'd rather avoid, such as examining painful family patterns, childhood wounds, and limiting beliefs that have been running your life from the shadows.

The Physical Dimension (Body)

Your body is a living, breathing miracle that responds to every thought, emotion, and spiritual experience you have. Every cell carries the memory of how you've treated it, how you've honored or neglected it, and how you've listened to or ignored its wisdom.

The physical dimension of healing goes far beyond taking the right supplements or following the perfect diet. Its focus is on developing a relationship with your body based on respect, gratitude, and partnership. When you understand your body as sacred—not in a religious sense necessarily, but as something worthy of reverence—everything changes.

Your cells begin to function differently when bathed in appreciation rather than criticism. Your digestive system works more efficiently when you eat with mindfulness rather than stress. Your immune system strengthens when you treat your body as a trusted ally rather than an enemy to be conquered.

I've witnessed patients whose chronic pain dissolved not through more aggressive treatment, but through learning to listen to what their bodies were trying to communicate. I've seen inflammatory markers normalize when people stopped fighting their symptoms and started honoring their body's need for rest, nourishment, and gentle movement.

The Spiritual Dimension (Spirit)

While religious practice provides a powerful framework for many people, the spiritual dimension is more about connecting to something greater than yourself, to your deepest values and the sacred nature of existence.

When this dimension is neglected, people often experience what I call "successful misery"—they achieve external markers of success while feeling empty, disconnected, and purposeless. Their bodies may function adequately, but they're not truly alive.

Spiritual health manifests as a sense of meaning in both joy and suffering, a connection to something beyond your immediate circumstances, and alignment between your daily choices and your deepest values. It's what gives you the strength to persevere through healing crises and the wisdom to make choices that serve your highest good rather than your immediate desires.

> **"For the simplicity that lies this side of complexity, I would not give a fig, but for the simplicity that lies on the other side of complexity, I would give my life."**
>
> OLIVER WENDELL HOLMES

These three dimensions don't operate independently; affecting one immediately influences the others, which is why purely physical approaches to chronic illness often fail, and why people who address only the psychological aspects without changing their lifestyle ultimately plateau in their healing.

Here is an illustrative case in point. David arrived at a local practice with severe digestive issues, chronic fatigue, and depression that had persisted for five years. He'd tried elimination diets, probiotics, and multiple rounds of antibiotics. He'd worked with therapists and tried various antidepressants. Nothing provided lasting relief.

During our comprehensive intake, a different picture emerged. David's symptoms had begun shortly after he'd taken a high-paying job that required him to compromise his ethical standards daily. The work paid well and impressed others, but it violated everything he believed about integrity and service.

His digestive system was literally rejecting this life choice. His fatigue reflected the enormous energy required to live in contradiction to his values. His depression was his soul's way of signaling that something was fundamentally wrong.

David's healing protocol included targeted nutrition and gut restoration, but the breakthrough came when he made the terrifying decision to leave his job and start a nonprofit organization aligned with his values. As his life came into integrity, his physical symptoms began to resolve. As he connected with his sense of purpose, his energy returned. As he aligned his daily actions with his spiritual convictions, his depression lifted.

This is what happens when you treat the whole person rather than isolated symptoms. Physical healing accelerates when it's supported by emotional clarity and spiritual alignment. Emotional breakthroughs become sustainable when they're grounded in physical practices and spiritual disciplines. Spiritual insights translate into lasting change when they're embodied in emotional intelligence and physical vitality.

Bridging Ancient Wisdom and Modern Science

Something remarkable is happening in healthcare. Rigid boundaries between science and spirituality—evidence-based medicine and faith-based healing—are beginning to dissolve. This is not because science is becoming less rigorous, but because it's becoming sophisticated enough to measure phenomena that were previously dismissed as unmeasurable.

The result is a new understanding that the most effective healing happens when ancient wisdom and modern science work together rather than in opposition. This integration expands our definition of what constitutes valid evidence. Consider the practice of regular meditation (some may use the term "prayer"), which literally rewires the brain, increasing activity in areas associated with attention and emotional regulation while decreasing activity in regions linked to anxiety and rumination.

Or take the concept of forgiveness, central to virtually every major spiritual tradition. Wise teachers have long claimed that forgiveness heals both the forgiver and the forgiven. Research now demonstrates that people who practice forgiveness have lower blood pressure, reduced chronic pain, improved immune function, and decreased risk of heart disease.[8]

The mechanisms are becoming clear. Resentment triggers a chronic stress response that floods the body with inflammatory chemicals. Forgiveness, however, activates the parasympathetic nervous system, shifting the body into repair mode.

Among the powerful drivers of this healing progression is faith as a measurable health factor. For example, people with active spiritual practices live longer, are generally happier, and are often more engaged in their communities.[9] The protective effect of spiritual practice is comparable to the difference between smoking and not smoking or exercising regularly and being sedentary.

But what exactly is it about spiritual practice—including meditation, prayer, and mindfulness—that promotes health? Several mechanisms are in play:[10]

Stress Reduction: Spiritual practices activate the relaxation response, normalizing cortisol levels and inflammatory markers. Prayer, meditation, and contemplative practices shift the nervous system out of fight-or-flight mode and into rest-and-repair mode.

Social Connection: Religious communities provide social support networks that are crucial for both mental and physical health.

Meaning-Making: Spiritual frameworks help people find meaning in suffering and purpose in daily life. This sense of meaning is powerfully protective against depression, anxiety, and even physical illness.

Comfort in Difficult Times: Most spiritual traditions provide guidance on navigating challenges such as illness, bereavement, unemployment, or relationship issues.

I've seen firsthand that when physical healing is supported by emotional clarity and spiritual alignment, it becomes not just more effective but more sustainable. Patients discover levels of vitality and purpose they never knew were possible.

I believe the future of medicine lies not in the replacement of science with spirituality, but the marriage of the two into something more powerful than either could be alone. It's healthcare that treats both the body and the soul, not just in the absence of disease but in the presence of extraordinary life.

PART TWO

Fundamental Principles of Foundational Health

Understanding chronic inflammation is just the beginning. Now we need to examine the core systems that fuel this inflammatory fire or help extinguish it entirely. These four interconnected systems—your gut, immune system, brain, and mitochondria—represent the biological foundation that determines whether you experience vibrant health or chronic struggle.

Think of these systems as the control centers of your body. When they function optimally, they create a powerful defense against the toxic bombardment we face daily. When they break down, they become the very mechanisms that perpetuate disease and accelerate aging.

In Chapter Four, we start with your gut—what experts call the "second brain" since it holds the key to virtually everything else. Your gut doesn't just digest food; it manufactures neurotransmitters that control your mood, houses much of your immune system, and serves as the gatekeeper that determines which substances enter your bloodstream. Central to this conversation is a permeable ("leaky") gut that triggers systemic inflammation, driving the likes of autoimmune conditions, brain fog, mood disorders, and countless other health problems. We'll go on to explore the critical gut-brain connection and its profound impact on mental health.

Chapter Five explores how gut dysfunction directly impacts your immune system, the furthest upstream cause of most chronic inflammatory diseases. We count on our immune systems to be powerful protectors, but when thrown off balance, they become our greatest threats, allowing chronic stress, poor sleep, and social isolation to derail a healthy body and healthy life. This chapter also looks closely at how to restore the immune system's proper function through targeted interventions.

Your brain and central nervous system are the focus of Chapter Seven. If your brain controls everything, how do you optimize it for peak performance? This chapter explores methods for optimizing the brain to perform at its highest potential, which goes on to augment longevity, cognitive function, and overall health quality.

Brains contain wildly intricate, highly functioning cells that manage much more than thinking and memory. Your brain controls hormone regulation, immune function, circadian rhythms, and every vital process keeping you alive. At its core is a remarkable capacity for neuroplasticity—your brain can literally rewire itself for better health at any age—but only if you provide the right conditions. We'll show you exactly how to optimize brain function through specific dietary choices, exercise protocols, and sleep strategies.

Finally, Chapter Eight addresses the cellular powerhouses themselves—your mitochondria. These microscopic energy factories determine whether you wake up energized or exhausted, whether your body can repair itself effectively, and whether you age gracefully or deteriorate rapidly. In fact, overall health is directly proportional to mitochondrial health, yet this element is often overlooked by physicians and largely unknown by patients.

This section is different from typical health advice, as we learn in detail that these systems don't function independently. Gut health directly influences immune responses, the immune system affects brain function, and the brain controls stress response, which impacts mitochondria, and back to the gut microbiome. And healthy mitochondria provide the energy needed for optimal gut, immune, and brain function.

It's all interconnected, and addressing symptoms in isolation rarely creates lasting change. For example, someone struggling with depression, digestive issues, frequent infections, and chronic fatigue isn't dealing with four separate problems—they're experiencing the downstream effects of dysfunction in foundational systems.

By understanding and optimizing these core systems as one, you can move beyond simply managing symptoms to restoring the biological resilience that allows your body to thrive. And that's where real transformation begins.

CHAPTER 4
Gut Health

All disease begins in the gut.
Hippocrates

It happens at the start line of a big race, a school presentation, the interview for your dream job, and random, glorious moments of love with someone special—that feeling of butterflies in your stomach. That's because your gut isn't just the place that digests your lunch; it's a byproduct of an intricate connection of trillions of microorganisms at work in your gut. In fact, the gut is often referred to as the "second brain," as it controls virtually every aspect of human health from immune response to mental clarity.

The digestive tract is home to a complex ecosystem working around the clock to maintain your health. This microscopic community—the gut microbiome—produces signaling molecules that travel throughout the body, promoting healing in ligaments, tendons, joints, the gut lining itself, and even brain tissue. When this system functions at full throttle, you thrive in similar fashion. If there's a chink in the armor, a cascade of health problems can follow.

How does it all work? Think of the gut microbiome as the command center for multiple critical body systems. At the controls is the vagus nerve, which runs from the brain to the large intestine and most everywhere in between. This extensive communication network maintains constant dialogue with your central nervous system, immune system, and other vital organs, including beneficial gut flora bacteria that support your body's natural healing processes. For example, one remarkable peptide, BPC-157 (Body Protective Compound 157), is produced in the gastric juices that travel throughout your body to signal repair and regeneration.

Nutrient absorption and metabolism also depend on gut flora. A balanced and diverse microbiome efficiently processes the foods you eat, extracting maximum nutritional value and converting dietary components into beneficial compounds your body needs. This optimal function then supports energy production at the cellular level, particularly in your mitochondria—your cells' powerhouses.

This interconnection between gut health and overall wellness is a big deal. Simply stated, a healthy gut acts as both a nutrient-processing center, a control center of sorts, and as a protective barrier, keeping beneficial substances in and harmful elements out. But what happens when the system breaks down?

The integrity of the gut lining is one of your body's most important and strongest defensive barriers. When functioning optimally, this membrane allows beneficial nutrients to pass through while blocking harmful substances. However, if the lining becomes compromised—a condition commonly known as "leaky gut"—serious health consequences can follow.

What is leaky gut syndrome? It occurs when the intestinal lining becomes abnormally permeable, allowing larger particles that would normally be blocked to pass through—things like undigested food components, microbes, and lipopolysaccharides (LPS), essentially toxic fragments that should remain contained within the digestive tract.

A breach of this protective barrier triggers an immediate immune response. Seventy percent of the body's immune cells surround the gut lining, standing guard against potential invaders. When these cells detect unwanted guests passing through the compromised barrier, they recognize the invasion and begin producing defensive antibodies.

This immune activation can lead to a state of chronic inflammation and autoimmune dysfunction, such as Hashimoto's thyroiditis, mentioned previously. For instance, a body with a compromised gut barrier may produce antibodies against gluten particles that have leaked through. But the antibodies don't discriminate between "good" and "bad." In a word, molecular mimicry essentially fakes out the immune system, as some thyroid cells appear similar to gluten proteins. In a case of mistaken identity, the body begins attacking its own thyroid tissue, leading to decreased hormone production and the eventual need for thyroid replacement therapy.

The inflammatory cascade triggered by leaky gut doesn't stop at autoimmune conditions. The compromised gut lining also mirrors the permeability of the blood-brain barrier, meaning that when your gut becomes leaky, your brain's protective barrier follows suit, often becoming compromised as well. This allows inflammatory particles to enter your central nervous system, potentially contributing to brain fog, mood disorders, hormonal dysregulation, and various neurological symptoms.

It's tough to defend against too, as leaky gut often begins with a single affront to the digestive system—food poisoning from travel, a course of antibiotics, chronic stress, or eating inflammatory foods. This damage can set off a domino effect that compromises the delicate balance of your gut microbiome and the integrity of your intestinal lining. For example, my untoward reaction to the antibiotic I took to assuage traveler's sickness adversely affected my mitochondrial function as well. For many weeks, I was profoundly weak and struggled just to get out of a chair.

In a related example, I'll share the story of AK, a thirty-eight-year-old woman who came to our practice for help. AK had a history of ulcerative colitis (an autoimmune inflammatory bowel condition), chronic fatigue, anxiety, insomnia, Hashimoto's thyroiditis with hypothyroidism, polycystic ovarian syndrome, and we have now diagnosed her with CIRS (chronic inflammatory response syndrome).

Her symptoms first manifested in her late teens, and she suffered with them for many years. Even after treating her for SIBO (small intestinal bacterial overgrowth—a common condition in those with leaky gut/autoimmune/CIRS-related conditions) and being on a strict autoimmune/anti-inflammatory diet, AK did not see significant improvement in her colitis symptoms. It wasn't until we started treating her with the peptide protocol for CIRS that she was finally free of her colitis symptoms. After four months of the CIRS treatment protocol with peptides, she felt better in all aspects except for the fatigue. Her inflammatory markers had all normalized within that time frame. AK's outlook and hope are now extremely positive. She plans to stay on a maintenance protocol, and we are hopeful that, with some additional strategies to enhance mitochondrial function, her chronic fatigue can be lifted as well.

In her case and mine, the road back to functional health starts from the inside.

Rebuilding Your Internal Ecosystem

The foundation of restoring and maintaining optimal gut health lies in nourishing beneficial microorganisms that call your digestive tract home. This means adopting a comprehensive approach that addresses diet, supplementation, and lifestyle factors.

It starts with nourishing the good flora. Beneficial gut bacteria thrive on specific types of nutrition, primarily prebiotics. Prebiotics are dietary fibers that act like fertilizer for your good bacteria, helping them flourish and outcompete harmful microorganisms. The most effective prebiotics come from foods—vegetables, herbs, and fruits—all the colorful stuff in your grocery store's produce section.

The foundation of a gut-healing diet should be built with vegetables to provide a diverse array of fibers required by different beneficial bacteria species. Herbs and seasonal fruits, for example, provide additional micronutrients and compounds that support microbial diversity. (It's worth noting that fruits, while loaded with beneficial nutrients, are essentially nature's candy and should be consumed in moderation compared to vegetables.)

Polyphenols represent another crucial category of gut-supporting compounds. These powerful antioxidants are found in foods like extra virgin olive oil (from quality sources), berries, dark leafy greens, and various herbs and spices. Polyphenols not only nourish beneficial bacteria but also help reduce inflammation throughout the digestive tract.

And we can't forget the power of fermentation. Before refrigeration revolutionized food storage, fermentation was humanity's primary method of food preservation (likely started by chance around 8,000 BCE with the storing of food in containers[11]). This ancient practice didn't just extend shelf life; it created incredibly beneficial foods that supported optimal gut health. Unfortunately, modern society has largely abandoned these traditional fermented foods, to our collective detriment.

Fermented vegetables like sauerkraut, kimchi, and real pickles (the kind that require refrigeration and contain live cultures) provide a powerful combination of beneficial microorganisms. These foods contain spore-based probiotics that originate from the soil, travel into the plants, and survive the fermentation process. These hardy organisms are particularly effective at healing the gut lining and can survive stomach acid better than many other probiotic strains.

Fermented dairy products like yogurt and kefir offer different strains of beneficial bacteria, contributing to microbial diversity. The key is choosing products that contain live, active cultures rather than processed versions that have been heat-treated. What makes fermented vegetables particularly special is that they provide both probiotics (the beneficial organisms themselves) and postbiotics (the beneficial compounds these organisms produce). During fermentation, good bacteria work overtime to produce substances called butyrates (postbiotics), which are incredibly healing and protective to the gut lining.

Keep in mind that while healthy food should always be the foundation of gut health, targeted supplementation can accelerate efficient healing and restoration. For example, I recommend a broad-spectrum, high-quality probiotic supplement to help reestablish beneficial bacteria populations, particularly after antibiotic use or during times of high stress. For those who wrinkle their nose at fermented veggies, I suggest taking spore-based probiotic supplements as well as other types of probiotics.

Prebiotic supplements can also be valuable, especially for individuals who struggle to consume adequate fiber from food sources. These supplements feed your existing beneficial bacteria and help newly introduced probiotics establish themselves in your gut ecosystem.

The timing and combination of supplements also play a big role. Taking prebiotics simultaneously with antibiotics can help offset much of the damage to gut flora caused by commercial medications, as prebiotics nourish beneficial bacteria while antibiotics eliminate both good and harmful microorganisms.

I recently completed a certification course in peptides, and a couple of the lectures included a pediatrician and cardiologist who talked about a study in which they simultaneously gave patients a prebiotic along with a commonly used antibiotic. The result offset the deleterious effects of altering the gut flora because as the good and bad microbes were killed off in the gut, the prebiotic nourished the good organisms.

It's not an easy task to resurrect gut health, so to speak, but we can do it.

Connecting to Mental Health on the Gut-Brain Highway

The relationship between your gut and brain extends far beyond the occasional "gut feeling" or stress-induced upset stomach. This connection represents a sophisticated, bidirectional communication system that profoundly influences mental health, cognitive function, and emotional well-being.

The gut-brain axis operates through multiple pathways, including the vagus nerve, immune system signals, and the production of neurotransmitters by gut bacteria. Fascinatingly, the gut microbiome produces many of the same neurotransmitters found in the brain, including serotonin, dopamine, and GABA (gamma-aminobutyric acid), a "calm down" neurotransmitter that blocks specific brain signals to help reduce anxiety, inspire relaxation and quality sleep, and balance mood swings. This means the health of your gut directly influences your brain's chemical environment.

When gut health is compromised, the effects on mental health can be swift and severe. Chronic inflammation in the gut triggers corresponding inflammation in the brain, as the integrity of the gut lining mirrors that of the blood-brain barrier. When inflammatory particles cross the blood-brain barrier into the central nervous system, they can disrupt the function of critical regulatory structures like the hypothalamus, pituitary gland, and pineal gland. This neuroinflammation can manifest as difficulty concentrating, depression, and hormonal imbalances. The traditional medical model often treats each of these as separate mental health issues, but they're symptoms of a much bigger problem—underlying gut dysfunction is commonly associated with immune and mitochondrial dysfunction. At its core, this reflects a single interconnected process—gut-driven inflammation impacting brain function and systemic regulation. Put simply, a troubled gut doesn't stay in the gut—it quickly becomes a troubled brain.

The gut-brain connection is why stress has such immediate and profound effects on digestive health. Chronic stress shifts the nervous system into a state of sympathetic dominance (fight-or-flight mode), which disrupts gut flora balance and can compromise intestinal barrier function. This creates a vicious cycle where gut dysfunction contributes to mental health symptoms, which increases stress and further damages gut health.

A full understanding of this connection underlines the importance of addressing mental health holistically. Rather than viewing psychological symptoms as purely brain-based issues, a comprehensive approach considers the gut as a primary treatment target for many mental health concerns.

But there is a dark side that must not be overlooked: modern medicine. While intensely promoted modern medications have undoubtedly saved countless lives, they have also become a societal pied piper, inspiring overuse and misuse to a widespread crisis of gut health dysfunction. Antibiotics, in particular, represent a double-edged sword that can devastate the delicate ecosystem of your gut microbiome.

Antibiotics are great at killing bacteria, but, as a general rule, they do not distinguish between beneficial and harmful microorganisms. A single course of broad-spectrum antibiotics such as Augmentin (unfortunately common practice for many people) can eliminate decades worth of carefully cultivated beneficial bacteria in your gut. This wholesale destruction can trigger a litany of health problems that persist long after the original infection has been treated.

And the damage often extends beyond bacterial elimination. Antibiotic exposure can lead to the overgrowth of opportunistic organisms like candida (yeast) and other harmful bacteria such as Clostridium difficile (often referred to as C. diff) that are often resistant to medication. These organisms "hide out" in the disrupted gut environment, waiting for their chance to further compromise digestive health and immune function.

Even worse, modern antibiotic exposure isn't limited to prescribed medications. A vivid example is the agricultural industry, which routinely feeds antibiotics to cattle, chickens, and other livestock, which means you are likely consuming antibiotic residues in meat, dairy products, and eggs. This chronic, low-level exposure can gradually erode gut health over time, casting a dimmer view on breakfast omelets and weekend burgers.

Beyond antibiotics, many common substances can disrupt gut health in ways most people never consider. Artificial sweeteners, particularly sucralose, act like antibiotics in the gut, destroying beneficial bacteria and altering the microbiome composition. Despite being marketed as "healthier" alternatives to sugar, these compounds can increase the risk of weight gain, insulin resistance, and type 2 diabetes by disrupting metabolic processes controlled by gut bacteria.

Even people who avoid artificial sweeteners often consume high-fructose corn syrup, a highly concentrated form of fructose that throws a wrench in the liver's natural processing capacities. This compound, found in multitudes of ingredients lists, can contribute to fatty liver disease, elevated uric acid levels, metabolic dysfunction, and gut health deterioration. Bad news on all fronts.

Arguably gravest on the list of health assaults are energy drinks, a particularly toxic combination of gut-disrupting substances containing high levels of caffeine, artificial sweeteners or high-fructose corn syrup, and various chemical additives. Billions of dollars are funneled into marketing these products to susceptible demographics, convinced they can go longer or faster by guzzling "energy" in a can. Some people even use these products to self-medicate conditions like ADHD or depression, while simultaneously damaging the gut health that is foundational to their mental wellness.

This circles back to how the blood-brain barrier mirrors gut integrity. We've been taught to believe that mental health is separate from physical and spiritual health. But it doesn't work that way. We are one being—one soul, all interconnected—very similar to the natural world in which we live. We no longer work *with* nature and are instead driven by modern society's penchant for lording over rather than living with the environment that sustains us. Exploiting resources for short-term use (often at the risk of extinction) leaves the whole in disarray. We must care for what's here now so it remains healthy as well and keeps providing. Holistic health works the same way.

Mental health is not separate from physical and spiritual health. We are one being—one soul, all interconnected—very similar to the natural world in which we live. We must care for the whole so it remains healthy and keeps providing.

Restoring Balance

There is a way out of the gut health blues and onto the track of a healthy, balanced life. First, remember that recovering from antibiotic damage or chronic gut dysfunction requires a comprehensive, patient approach. The good news is that the gut has a remarkable healing capacity when given proper support and conditions.

Immediately after antibiotic exposure, aggressive probiotic supplementation becomes crucial. This means using broad-spectrum, high-potency probiotic supplements that contain multiple strains of beneficial bacteria. Equally important is supplementing with prebiotics to nourish beneficial flora ("good gut buddies," as Dr. Steven Gundry says). The goal is to quickly reestablish microbial diversity and prevent harmful organisms from colonizing the disrupted gut environment.

For the long term, a selection of lifestyle approaches can stimulate the parasympathetic side, the rest and digest side, of the autonomic nervous system:

Stress Management: Chronic stress represents one of the most significant threats to gut health. Stress-reduction practices like meditation, breathing exercises that promote carbon dioxide retention, or therapeutic touch can help shift the nervous system into parasympathetic dominance, which supports optimal gut function.

Sleep Optimization: Quality sleep is absolutely critical for gut health recovery. During sleep, your body performs essential repair and maintenance functions, including gut lining regeneration and microbiome rebalancing. Poor sleep quality, on the other hand, can quickly undo progress made through dietary and supplemental interventions. We will touch on this later, but the peptide Epitalon is magic for restoring our circadian rhythm through the pineal gland.

Cold Therapy: Controlled cold exposure, such as cold-water immersion, can help reset the autonomic nervous system and support overall healing processes. This practice stimulates the parasympathetic nervous system (after temporarily stimulating the sympathetic side) and may enhance the body's natural repair mechanisms. Try wrapping up your shower with a minute or two of cold water to improve circulation, boost your energy, and help build resilience to stress.

Advanced Interventions: In cases of severe gut dysfunction, additional therapeutic approaches may be necessary. This is where peptide therapy comes in, directly supporting gut lining repair and other targeted interventions that can address specific aspects of digestive dysfunction.

Remember that the recovery process is rarely quick or simple. Depending on the degree of damage and dysfunction, healing may take months or (rarely) years of consistent effort. However, with persistence and the right approach, significant improvement is not only possible but expected.

The importance of gut health cannot be overestimated. If we don't prioritize it, we simply cannot expect to be optimally healthy. Your gut controls or significantly influences virtually every aspect of your physiology. And this is far more than just improving digestion or addressing specific symptoms; it establishes the foundation for optimal health throughout your entire life, in potent, visible ways.

One of the impactful benefits of a healthy gut microbiome is optimal mitochondrial function, which directly impacts your energy levels and cellular health; in reality, every aspect of your health. Signaling molecules produced by beneficial bacteria help coordinate healing and repair processes throughout your body, from your joints and muscles to your brain and cardiovascular system. Proper gut health that maximizes the nutritional value of everything you consume while minimizing the absorption of harmful substances also optimizes nutrient absorption and utilization. No matter how healthy your diet, if your gut cannot properly process and absorb nutrients as well as send critical signals to the mitochondria, brain and elsewhere, you cannot achieve optimal health.

Perhaps most importantly, optimal gut health serves as a powerful defense against chronic disease. A balanced microbiome supports proper immune function, reduces systemic inflammation, and helps maintain the integrity of protective barriers throughout your body. Ultimately, stalwart foundational health makes you more resilient against infections, autoimmune conditions, metabolic disorders, and even certain cancers.[12]

At the risk of "grossing the reader out," one of the treatment modalities that I employed when I was so desperately ill after my severe untoward reaction to the antibiotic Cipro was that of a fecal microbiota transplant. That's right! My microbiome had virtually been wiped out, and I had to start from scratch. I borrowed stool samples from a young healthy male athlete, processed them, and used them via enema to help reestablish flora. Unfortunately, in the United States it is only approved for treating resistant Clostridium difficile colitis, except in research settings. I do not recommend people do this without medical supervision, but I will say it was one of the many things that helped restore my gut and overall health.

All told, understanding gut health requires embracing a holistic view of human wellness. I've emphasized how our bodies operate as integrated systems where every component influences all the others around it. Conventional medical approaches often treat symptoms in isolation, addressing mental health separately from physical health and viewing each organ system as independent. But that's not how we're wired. The reality of human physiology demands a more integrated approach that recognizes the gut as the central hub connecting *all* aspects of health. There is very good reason that "health in the navel" is mentioned first in the list of blessings from the God-given health code mentioned earlier.

When you prioritize gut health, you make an investment in your energy levels, mental clarity, immune function, hormonal balance, and long-term disease resistance. You're working *with* your body's natural healing mechanisms. In our culture of quick fixes and immediate gratification, this perspective requires patience and a long-term mindset. Yes, gut health recovery can seem frustratingly slow, but the investment pays dividends for decades to come. Someone who prioritizes gut health in their thirties and forties often enjoys vibrant health well into their eighties and nineties, while those who neglect this foundation may struggle with chronic health issues much earlier in life.

Your gut truly is your second brain. By recognizing its central role in your overall health and taking concrete steps to optimize its function, you're not just improving one aspect of your wellness; you are transforming your entire health trajectory.

CHAPTER 5

Immune Health

The body is a self-healing organism, so it's really about clearing things out of the way so the body can heal itself.

Barbara Brennan

When talking about autoimmune disease, my patients frequently think that it just means an overactive immune system. That's true to a degree, but when one side of the immune system is overactive, typically the other side is underactive. Your immune system does a lot more than you think. It's in control of many aspects of our health, locating, chaperoning, and addressing problems early on with built-in checks and balances. When this system is not in balance, it opens a door for chronic inflammatory processes.

Unfortunately, laypeople, and even those in the medical community, have been led to believe that our immune system is either overactive, underactive, or right where it should be. But it's much more complex than that.

Here's a closer look: Your immune system operates as a complex surveillance network designed to protect you from countless threats, yet its success hinges on an unexpected alliance with your digestive tract. This partnership represents one of biology's most sophisticated relationships, where microscopic organisms in your intestines directly influence your body's defensive capabilities.

The intestinal tract is your body's primary immune headquarters, perfectly positioned to do its thing. The digestive system is the main gateway through which external substances enter your internal environment. Every morsel of food, every beverage, every supplement must pass through this checkpoint, where specialized immune cells evaluate whether incoming materials pose threats or provide benefits.

Within this environment lives the gut microbiome, a vast ecosystem containing trillions of microorganisms that have coexisted with humans throughout evolutionary history. These microscopic inhabitants actively participate in immune education, teaching your defensive cells how to distinguish between dangerous invaders and harmless visitors. When functioning optimally, this microbial community guides immune responses with remarkable precision.

A thriving microbiome produces metabolites that strengthen intestinal walls, creating a selective barrier that welcomes nutrients while blocking harmful substances. These beneficial compounds nourish the cells that line your gut, maintaining tight connections between them. This selective permeability allows your body to absorb essential nutrients while preventing toxins and pathogens from entering your bloodstream.

However, contemporary lifestyle factors consistently undermine this delicate relationship. Ultra-processed foods lacking adequate fiber deprive beneficial microbes of necessary nutrients. Chemical additives and preservatives can directly harm microbial populations. Medical interventions, while sometimes essential, may disrupt bacterial communities for extended periods. Persistent stress produces hormones that alter microbial composition and weaken intestinal barriers.

Immune Dysregulation

When microbial balance shifts—creating what researchers term dysbiosis—the repercussions extend throughout your entire system. Opportunistic bacteria may multiply, releasing inflammatory substances that activate immune responses inappropriately. The intestinal barrier may become compromised, permitting bacterial components and partially digested materials to cross into circulation, where they trigger widespread inflammatory reactions.

When that happens, your immune system may begin responding excessively or targeting inappropriate substances. This dysregulation can manifest as heightened sensitivity to foods, environmental substances, or even your own tissues, which can go on to trigger the nervous system to react with altered mood, concentration difficulties, or persistent exhaustion.

Case Study: Functional Medicine Approach to Immune Dysregulation

PATIENT PROFILE

Age/Sex: 29-year-old female

Presenting Complaints: Chronic diarrhea-predominant irritable bowel syndrome (IBS-D), recurrent headaches, brain fog, premenstrual dysphoria, persistent fatigue, and plaque psoriasis.

History: Symptoms had been ongoing for several years with significant impact on daily functioning, mood, and quality of life. Conventional treatments (symptomatic medications, dermatologic creams, oral contraceptives) provided limited or temporary relief.

FUNCTIONAL MEDICINE ASSESSMENT

Key Findings

- Evidence of immune dysregulation (elevated inflammatory markers, low natural killer cell activity, elevated transforming growth factor beta 1, and a low melanocyte-stimulating hormone level).
- Gut dysbiosis and increased intestinal permeability on stool/functional testing (and a matrix metalloproteinase 9 level of over 1,000).
- Elevated hs-CRP and borderline anti-nuclear antibody, though not diagnostic for systemic autoimmune disease.
- Hormonal fluctuations contributing to cyclical mood changes.
- Poor sleep architecture with lack of deep and REM sleep

Clinical Interpretation

The constellation of IBS-D, brain fog, psoriasis, insomnia, and fatigue was understood through the lens of immune dysregulation driving systemic inflammation, worsened by impaired gut barrier function and neuroendocrine imbalance.

THERAPEUTIC INTERVENTIONS

1. **Pharmacologic/Peptide Support**
   - Low-Dose Naltrexone (LDN): To modulate immune activity and reduce neuroinflammation.
   - Immunomodulating Peptides (e.g., Thymogen alpha-1 [Integrative Peptides branded], TB4 Frag): Targeted at restoring immune homeostasis and supporting gut mucosal healing. Optimizing omega -3 fatty acid levels, phospholipids, and curcuminoids.
2. **Gut-Healing Protocol**
   - Autoimmune Protocol (AIP) Diet: Elimination of gluten, dairy (but allowing for A2 casein-derived dairy), processed foods, and inflammatory triggers.
   - Targeted Nutraceuticals: Prebiotic fiber, spore-based probiotics/fermented veggies, BPC 157, and postbiotics/tributyrin to restore barrier integrity.
3. **Lifestyle & Functional Support**
   - Optimized sleep hygiene and circadian alignment through supplementing with Epitalon for a one-month reset.
   - Stress regulation techniques (yoga, mindfulness, breathwork).
   - Gradual increase in exercise to support mitochondrial function and energy balance along with other mitochondrial enhancement strategies.

OUTCOMES (AFTER SIX MONTHS)

Symptomatic Improvements

- Diarrhea resolved; bowel regularity restored.
- Headaches and brain fog markedly diminished.

- Premenstrual mood disturbances resolved.
- Psoriasis cleared with no new lesions.
- Energy improved dramatically—transition from chronic fatigue to sustained vitality.
- Sleep became deeper and restorative.

Biomarker Improvements

- hs-CRP, ESR, and other inflammatory markers normalized.
- Reduction in intestinal permeability markers.
- Improved cortisol rhythm on salivary testing.

DISCUSSION

This case highlights the role of a functional medicine approach in addressing chronic, multi-system symptoms rooted in immune dysregulation. Conventional care had been insufficient, but by integrating LDN, immunomodulatory peptides, sleep restoration, and gut-directed therapies within an anti-inflammatory dietary framework, the patient achieved significant clinical remission. Importantly, the restoration of gut and immune balance not only improved physical symptoms but also resolved mood instability and fatigue—leading to a renewed sense of health and vitality.

Rebounding from this scenario is particularly challenging. While microbial imbalance disrupts immune function, immune hyperactivity further damages the gut environment, establishing a self-reinforcing cycle. Ongoing inflammation transforms the intestinal environment, promoting harmful microbes while suppressing beneficial ones, creating increasingly inhospitable conditions.

Where does that leave us? Recognizing this interconnection transforms our approach to immune wellness. Rather than addressing immune challenges as isolated problems requiring separate solutions, we can focus on supporting gut health as a pathway to immune equilibrium. This involves prioritizing foods that nourish beneficial microbes, reducing inflammatory triggers, and sometimes implementing targeted strategies to restore microbial diversity and repair intestinal integrity.

The partnership between your immune system and gut microbiome exemplifies biological cooperation in action. When this alliance functions harmoniously, it provides robust protection while maintaining internal balance to achieve lasting immune resilience and overall vitality.

One way I explain this concept to my patients is with a scenario involving an initial insult to the gut lining, such as the severe traveler's diarrhea I brought home from Mexico. Here's what happens: Even after the acute symptoms resolve (the diarrhea clears up in four to five days, for example), damage to the gut lining often persists. This compromised barrier allows microbes and food particles to pass through into the bloodstream—the "leaky gut" condition we discussed earlier.

When these foreign substances breach the gut barrier, the immune system immediately springs into action. It's designed to identify and neutralize these invaders, but this constant state of alert can push the immune system into overdrive. Over time, in susceptible individuals, this leads to a critical imbalance where the regulatory side (TH1 or T-helper cells) becomes underactive while the inflammatory side (TH2 or TH17 cells) becomes overactive. This imbalance creates a state of chronic inflammation that becomes self-perpetuating.

Once this immune dysfunction takes hold, inflammation goes unchecked, and a cascade of health problems begins. These "falling dominoes" manifest differently in each person, largely determined by individual genetic makeup and predispositions. The result is often a constellation of chronic health issues that can seem unrelated but stem from this fundamental gut-immune imbalance.

While gut damage often initiates this cycle, the relationship between gut and immune health is bidirectional. Sometimes immune dysfunction comes first through viral infections such as COVID-19, vaccine reactions in genetically predisposed individuals, or environmental toxins like mold exposure. When the immune system becomes imbalanced from these non-gut insults, the compromised immune function can then damage gut tissue, creating the same problematic cycle from the opposite direction.

Whether it starts with gut damage leading to immune dysfunction, or immune problems causing gut issues, the end result is the same: a self-reinforcing cycle of inflammation and tissue damage that can manifest as various chronic health conditions. Understanding this bidirectional relationship is crucial for effective treatment and recovery.

Immune Dysfunction Triggers

Can there be other influences on immune function? Most certainly. Triggers that can set off immune dysfunction extend far beyond physical insults to the gut. Emotional and psychological factors play a surprisingly significant role, demonstrating the deep interconnection of mental, emotional, and physical health.

For instance, emotional trauma represents one of the most under-recognized yet powerful prompts of immune imbalance. The death of a loved one, personal trauma, or ongoing abuse situations can create profound physiological changes in the body that launch the same cascade of immune dysfunction as physical insults.

Here's what happens: When we experience acute trauma, our bodies respond by initially increasing cortisol production. As the condition persists and becomes chronic, we will often underproduce cortisol, which then exacerbates the inflammation and contributes to lethargy and fatigue. Even relatively short periods of poor, non-restorative sleep can be sufficient to trigger immune system imbalance in susceptible individuals.

The connection between stress and gut health is particularly striking. Research demonstrates that stress immediately and directly compromises the integrity of the gut lining. This means that emotional trauma can create the same leaky gut condition that we see from physical insults, setting off the identical cycle of immune dysfunction and chronic inflammation.

Beyond emotional triggers, numerous other factors can overwhelm the immune system and create lasting imbalance:

Environmental toxins, such as chronic exposure to heavy metals, pesticides, biotoxins, and industrial chemicals, can gradually erode immune function.

Poor nutrition, particularly diets high in processed foods and sugar while lacking essential nutrients, creates a state of chronic low-grade inflammation that stresses the immune system over time.

Hormonal imbalances, whether from thyroid dysfunction, reproductive hormone disruption, use of hormonal contraception, or adrenal fatigue, can also significantly impact immune regulation. That's because the endocrine and immune systems are closely intertwined, with hormones serving as important signaling molecules that help coordinate immune responses.

Chronic infections that persist under the radar—such as viral reactivation of Epstein-Barr virus, cytomegalovirus, or chronic bacterial infections like Lyme disease—can keep the immune system in a constant state of imbalance. This ongoing immune dysregulation can eventually lead to the same TH1/TH2 imbalance we see with chronic inflammation.

Physical trauma is a big deal as well. Surgeries, accidents, or chronic physical stress from overexercise or poor ergonomics create inflammatory responses that can overwhelm the body's ability to return to balance. Even seemingly minor physical stresses, when chronic, can accumulate to create significant immune dysfunction.

Adding to all this, our modern lifestyle presents multiple simultaneous challenges to immune function. Disrupted circadian rhythms from artificial light exposure and irregular sleep schedules, social isolation, chronic work stress, and constant stimulation from technology all contribute to a state of chronic physiological stress that can trigger immune imbalance and open the door to unchecked chronic inflammation.

The key insight is that immune dysfunction rarely results from a single cause. Instead, it typically emerges from the accumulation of multiple stressors—physical, emotional, environmental, genetic predisposition, and lifestyle factors—that overwhelm the body's natural resilience and adaptive capacity. Understanding this multifactorial nature is crucial for both prevention and treatment, as it suggests that effective healing often requires addressing multiple dimensions of health simultaneously.

"I Never Get Sick"

One point I frequently address with my patients involves a common misconception about immune health. When discussing immune dysfunction, my patients often respond with, "But I never get sick." We need to be careful how we interpret this statement because it may not indicate what people think it does, especially if the patient experiences symptoms of chronic inflammation and immune dysregulation.

In some cases, "never getting sick" actually suggests that the immune system is compromised and out of balance. When the immune system is weak in certain aspects, we may not be mounting the appropriate immune response to insults that we should. A well-functioning immune system should occasionally recognize threats and respond accordingly. Never getting sick isn't necessarily a sign of optimal immune function—rather, it might indicate that the system isn't responding as it should.

What This Really Means

While you might go through your day feeling great and believing everything is functioning as it should, this doesn't necessarily mean that everything in your body is running perfectly. It's normal and expected to periodically get sick—perhaps a flu every few years where you mount a fever as the body attempts to fight off the infection. But when this *never* happens year after year, such as someone who never experiences a flu with a fever, it is ultimately unhealthy.

Just as building tolerance through exercise or hard work strengthens the body, getting sick occasionally allows your immune system to build toughness and resilience. I've jokingly expressed the motto: If you want a strong immune system, don't wash your hands; lick doorknobs. While obviously this is not literal medical advice, the underlying principle is important—we need exposure to pathogens to build a healthy natural immune response.

Research consistently supports this concept. Studies show that children in daycare settings initially get sick more often,[13] and pediatricians get sick more frequently when they first start medical practice. However, after this initial period of increased illness, both eventually develop stronger immune systems because they've been exposed to various pathogens and have properly trained their systems to respond.

This principle helps explain why we have such an increased incidence of atopic diseases like eczema, asthma, and allergies—we've become *too* clean. We all need outdoor exposure to diverse environments. We need to get dirty, to literally eat dirt sometimes, because this is how we develop a varied microbiome and properly train our immune systems. But society hasn't embraced this understanding, and I believe this approach compromises our health when all we do is try to avoid microbes at all costs.

The Mental and Emotional Aspects of Immune Function

The mental and emotional aspects of immune function are equally fascinating and powerful. I've known people who, when they feel a cold coming on, consciously tell themselves "I don't want to get sick" and actively channel that energy into their bodies to fight it off. And it worked.

The mind has a significant impact on the immune system, and this isn't just wishful thinking—there's solid science behind it.[14]

Decades ago, I read that hypnosis was the most successful treatment for viral warts. This finding is particularly interesting when you consider how we typically treat warts. These viruses survive on the skin's surface in areas with poor blood flow and limited vascular supply. Conventional treatments work by irritating the area—we freeze, burn, scrape, or apply caustic substances to stimulate the immune system to recognize the virus and produce antibodies against it.

But the mind can control this process as well. I've had success treating warts in my own children simply by applying Whiteout to them. I don't believe the Whiteout itself causes any therapeutic reaction, but it makes them *believe* the treatment works. This demonstrates the remarkable power of the placebo effect and the mind's influence over immune function.

The mind-body connection in immune health is one of the most underutilized aspects of medicine.

This isn't just psychological trickery—it represents a genuine physiological response where belief and expectation create measurable changes in immune function, inflammation, and healing. This mind-body connection in immune health is one of the most underutilized aspects of medicine, yet it offers profound implications for how we approach both prevention and treatment of immune-related conditions.

Understanding these principles—that occasional illness can be healthy, that exposure builds resilience, and that the mind powerfully influences immune function—fundamentally changes how we think about immune health and opens new possibilities for supporting our body's natural defensive capabilities.

Natural Immunity

The fallback treatment in today's medical community is: There's a pill for that. But is it the right one? Our instinct to immediately suppress symptoms or attack infections with medications often works against the body's natural learning processes. Each time the immune system successfully fights off an infection, it becomes better equipped to handle similar challenges in the future. When we consistently intervene with medications, we rob the immune system of these important training opportunities.

Consider children's pediatrics, with ear infections in particular. When a parent brings a child in with an earache, they expect to receive an antibiotic prescription. However, this isn't necessarily the best treatment approach. Research shows that approximately 80 percent of ear infections in children will resolve on their own without any intervention or treatment.[15] Most of these infections are viral, making antibiotics completely ineffective anyway.

More concerning is the evidence that when we do intervene and treat ear infections with antibiotics, children are more likely to develop recurrent ear infections compared to simply letting the infection run its course naturally. By allowing the body to fight off the infection on its own, the child develops natural immunity against similar future infections. The antibiotic intervention might seem helpful in the short term, but ultimately interferes with the natural immune development process.

This example represents a broader problem in how we approach minor illnesses, and the implications extend beyond just ear infections. This same principle applies to many common childhood illnesses and minor infections. While there are certainly times when medical intervention is necessary and appropriate, we've swung too far toward the interventionist approach, even for conditions that the body is perfectly capable of handling on its own.

Understanding these principles—that occasional illness can be healthy, that exposure builds resilience, that the mind powerfully influences immune function, and that medical intervention isn't always better than natural healing (I would venture to say that natural healing and natural immunity is almost always preferred)—fundamentally changes how we think about immune health and opens new possibilities for supporting our body's natural defensive capabilities.

All told, we can boost our immune systems naturally on three stages: lifestyle, nutrition, and supplements.

Lifestyle

Lifestyle is a broad-stroke topic, subjective to as many people as it is in connotation. When it comes to immune function, we must start with the fundamentals. Just as with physical health, proper restorative sleep is absolutely critical—not just for immune function, but for maintaining the integrity of our gut lining and overall health. Sleep is when our body performs its most crucial repair work, consolidating memories, clearing metabolic waste from the brain (glymphatic drainage), and allowing our immune system to reset and strengthen.

Exercise

Exercise represents another cornerstone of immune health, providing a powerful positive impact on our immune system.[16] Roughly sixty minutes of moderate to vigorous activity each day, or several days per week, brings the most immune-boosting benefits and stronger metabolic systems. However, like many good things, we can take it too far.[17] Extreme endurance exercise and associated overtraining can have the opposite effect by suppressing your immune system. For example, endurance athletes who fall into the trap of overtraining and under-recovery often find themselves with suppressed immune systems that make them more susceptible to illness and injury. I speak from personal experience here—my own pattern of overtraining and inadequate recovery contributed significantly to my degenerative disc disease and subsequent back surgeries. This was compounded by a chronic inflammation that I wasn't even aware of at the time. (If I had known then what I know now! For the endurance athlete out there, we now have strategies to mitigate that damage using sleep and healing peptides, hyperbaric oxygen recovery strategies, common sense, and more.)

Nutrition

Incorporating healthy nutrition is, of course, key to immune health as well. But what are the "right" things to eat? While certain foods and nutraceuticals can have direct positive effects on immune function, I believe the most significant impact of our diet comes through its influence on our gut microbiome, which in turn profoundly affects immune system balance and function.

Our primary goal should be nourishing the gut microbiome, and this happens primarily through plant fibers (and the avoidance of inflammatory foods, namely refined carbohydrates, inflammatory grains, and seed oils) and specifically vegetable and fruit fibers. These fibers serve as fuel for beneficial bacteria, allowing them to flourish and maintain the delicate ecosystem that supports our immune system. We should also be consuming probiotic-rich foods to introduce beneficial microbes into our systems. But remember, it's not enough to just consume probiotics—we must also augment them with the right fibers to help them establish and thrive.

VEGETABLES AND FRUIT

You'll notice I consistently mention vegetables before fruits, and this is intentional. I recommend to my patients a four-to-one ratio of vegetables to fruits. While fruits are nature's dessert and naturally appealing due to their sweetness (it's hard to resist gobbling pineapples, mangos, and dates), overconsumption can create problems, primarily due to the high fructose content in fruit.

This doesn't mean fruits are inherently bad—quite the opposite. The key is choosing wisely and consuming appropriately. Less sweet fruits with lower fructose content are generally better choices. Berries, kiwi, grapefruit, and green bananas, for example, offer tremendous nutritional value without the excessive sugar load that comes with many other fruits.

THE WISDOM OF SEASONALITY

There is profound wisdom in eating seasonally and locally. Good evidence suggests that consuming locally produced, seasonally fresh produce is superior for our health. This concept isn't new—it's reflected in ancient wisdom traditions and scriptures.

Consider the pattern described in the Word of Wisdom scripture: herbs and fruits "in the season thereof" are mentioned first, followed by "meat sparingly," with the clarification that this might not apply "in times of winter and famine." This revelation, given hundreds of years ago, reflects a deep understanding of nutritional needs across seasons.

During times of abundance—such as harvest season—we have access to a tremendous variety of plants, vegetables, and fruits. When we consume this diverse palette of produce, our nutritional needs are largely met, and we don't necessarily require much animal protein. This supports the principle of consuming meat sparingly.

However, there are natural exceptions. During colder months, when fresh produce was scarce, people historically turned to stored grains and preserved meats like elk jerky to sustain themselves through harsh winters. This seasonal adaptation makes perfect biological sense.

I believe there's intentional significance in listing herbs (referring generally to vegetables) and fruits first in this hierarchy. This represents the foundation of our nutritional pyramid—we need abundant plant foods. But I avoid the term "plant-based diet" because it often implies exclusion of animal products, which does not align with optimal health or divine design. Rather, we need substantial amounts of vegetables and fruits for their fibers, polyphenols, and other molecules that nourish our gut microbiome and support immune function.

Another powerful lesson from ancient peoples is that they consumed whatever nature provided in their specific region and season. Nature essentially provided the ideal diet for their circumstances and needs. We would benefit today from thinking more about the geography, seasonality, and climate of where we live as the lens through which to view our food choices. (That would likely represent a more ideal dietary pattern than Cheetos and Diet Coke—and supermarkets full of other processed foods that dominate modern diets.)

PROTEIN

Now, what about protein? Formed from the Greek word protos (meaning "first"), protein consumption is one of today's most misunderstood aspects of nutrition. Almost everywhere you look, the message is to ingest as much protein as possible. Typical recommendations circulating today—such as consuming a gram of protein per pound of body weight daily—are simply not founded on solid science. In fact, many of these recommendations often stem from bodybuilding culture and supplement marketing (the supplements industry spends billions every year to convince you of this[18]) rather than longevity research.

The truth is that for optimal health and longevity, substantial research suggests we don't need nearly as much protein as commonly believed. The recommended daily allowance for adult protein intake is just 0.36 grams per pound of body weight to maintain basic nutritional requirements. (That said, anyone engaged in resistance exercise should consider increasing protein intake by 50 percent, and any adult over age sixty, whether they're able to participate in resistance exercise or not.)

However, all things in moderation, correct? Our bodies efficiently recycle and reuse protein when dietary protein intake is moderate, reducing our external protein requirements. Study after study from longevity experts consistently shows that we need to limit protein intake for optimal health and longevity. While we certainly don't want to become protein-deficient, we must recognize that excessive protein consumption is not beneficial and can actually harm our health. The key is finding the optimal amount—enough to meet our needs without the negative consequences of overconsumption.

CHAPTER 6

The Supplement Foundation

The body will heal itself when given the right nutrients in the right amounts—our task is to identify what is missing.

Jeffrey Bland, PhD

While a balanced diet and restorative sleep remain the bedrock (pun intended) of immune health, targeted supplementation can provide crucial support when our bodies face increased demands or nutritional gaps. With the immune system operating as a complex network requiring specific vitamins, minerals, and compounds to function optimally, modern food processing, soil depletion, lifestyle stressors, and genetic factors (such as mthfr mutations, the gene that provides instructions for making an enzyme, one that plays a crucial role in processing vitamin B9 and converting it into its active form) often leave us deficient in key nutrients.

Supplements can fill critical gaps that even well-intentioned diets may miss. However, they work best as part of a comprehensive approach that addresses diet, lifestyle, genetic, and environmental factors. Understanding which nutrients directly support immune pathways, and how certain foods can either strengthen or sabotage these systems, empowers us to make informed decisions about our health.

The goal isn't to rely on supplements as a cure-all, but to use them strategically alongside immune-supporting foods while avoiding those that compromise our body's natural defenses. We also must keep a close eye on common dietary components that can significantly undermine immune system effectiveness:

Foods To Avoid

Ultra-Processed Foods, Refined Sugars, and Carbohydrates: Many packaged snacks, chips (the exception might be certain chips cooked in healthier oils that tolerate heat, such as avocado oil), candy, instant foods, most frozen pizzas, and foods high in additives. Obviously the list is far too long. Processed sugars and refined carbohydrates create inflammatory responses that suppress immune cell function for hours after consumption. These foods also feed harmful bacteria in the gut, disrupting the delicate balance needed for optimal immune function. In a very real sense, we are what we eat, and we are what we feed our microbiome, the conductor of much of our health symphony.

Processed and Fried Foods: Some fried foods and processed meats contain advanced glycation end products (AGEs) and other inflammatory compounds that burden the immune system and promote chronic inflammation.

Seed Oils: Industrial seed oils—including canola, soy, corn, sunflower, and safflower oils—may be equally detrimental to health as refined carbohydrates. These highly processed oils contain damaged fatty acids that integrate into cellular and mitochondrial membranes, stiffening these critical structures and reducing their efficiency. Resulting cellular damage compromises mitochondrial health and energy production, which directly impacts immune system function since immune cells require substantial energy to operate effectively. This really is a BIG deal. They simply wreak havoc on cellular health. Avoid them like the plague and politic to have them banned.

Excessive Alcohol: While moderate alcohol consumption may be claimed to have some benefits (and this claim is rife with debate), excessive intake suppresses immune cell activity and disrupts gut barrier function, making the body more susceptible to infections. All of the newest evidence suggests tha no alcohol is best.

In addition to avoiding these harmful foods, we can turn to a host of vitamins, minerals, and other dietary addendums that shape energy-rich, whole-body health.

Immune Support

Conceptually, we need to consider getting back to "traditional eating." Solid research conducted many decades ago has shown that traditional eating (think 100 or more years ago before the introduction of refined carbohydrates, sugar, seed oils, and mass agriculture) is leaps and bounds better for our foundational health. Consider the work done by Dr. Weston A. Price and his classic book, *Nutrition and Physical Degeneration*,[19] which showed that traditional, whole food diets produce robust health, while modern processed foods cause decay, disease, and degeneration. The Weston Price Foundation advocates whole, unprocessed foods, raw dairy, fermented foods, and properly prepared ancient grains.

Quality Proteins: Provide amino acids essential for antibody production and immune cell maintenance.

Fatty Fish: Omega-3 fatty acids that regulate inflammation and support immune cell communication. (The acronym SMASH helps us remember which are the smaller cold water fatty fish: Salmon, Mackerel, Anchovies, Sardines, and Herring.)

Nuts and Seeds: Offer healthy fats, vitamin E, and minerals crucial for immune function (one example is the selenium content in Brazil nuts).

Probiotic-Rich Foods: Fermented foods like sauerkraut, kimchi, yogurt, and kefir directly support beneficial gut bacteria.

Premium Olive Oil

High-quality, bitter olive oils—particularly those from California, Morocco, and other Mediterranean regions—contain exceptional levels of polyphenols. These powerful antioxidants provide significant immune system benefits by reducing oxidative stress and supporting anti-inflammatory pathways. The bitter taste indicates higher polyphenol content, making these oils particularly valuable for gut/immune support.

Key Immune-Supporting Supplements

ESSENTIAL VITAMINS AND MINERALS

In the world of vitamins and minerals, the key is a comprehensive approach to immune support, including these key nutrients:

Vitamin A: Critical for maintaining mucous membrane integrity and supporting immune cell differentiation.

B-Complex Vitamins (B6, Folate, B12): Essential for immune cell production and function.

Vitamin C: Powerful antioxidant that supports white blood cell function and collagen synthesis.

Vitamin D: Regulates immune system response and has anti-inflammatory properties.

Vitamin K: Supports immune system regulation and bone health and, to a degree, even cardiovascular health.

Zinc: Plays a crucial role in killing intracellular microbes and supporting immune cell development. It's particularly important for wound healing and maintaining the integrity of skin and mucous membranes.

SUPPORTING MINERALS

Copper: Works synergistically with zinc for immune function.

Iodine: Essential for thyroid function, which influences immune system activity.

Iron: Necessary for immune cell proliferation and function (a word of caution, however—we do not want to have excess iron, as it contributes to oxidative stress).

Magnesium: Supports over 300 enzymatic reactions, many involved in immune function. (We could write a book just on the topic of this marvelous mineral.)

Selenium: Powerful antioxidant that protects immune cells from oxidative damage.

The common thread in immune system health, and the most effective strategy, is a nutrient-dense, whole foods diet blended with targeted supplementation. Rather than relying solely on supplements, focus on creating a foundation of immune-supporting foods while using high-quality supplements to fill specific gaps or provide additional support during times of increased stress or exposure risk. Remember, they are called supplements for a very good reason—they supplement, not replace, an optimal diet.

Immune Dysfunction

Among its importance to overall health and inherent intricacies of operation, an imbalanced immune system can open the door for a variety of problems:

1. Chronic inflammation
    - Persistent activation of cytokines
    - Ongoing fatigue, malaise, pain, and tissue damage
    - Low-grade systemic inflammation that drives aging (inflammaging)
2. Autoimmunity
    - Immune system attacks self-tissues
    - Examples include Hashimoto's thyroiditis, rheumatoid arthritis, lupus, multiple sclerosis, type 1 diabetes, and more
3. Immune Suppression/Susceptibility to Infection (usually chronic)
    - Paradoxical effect: immune system is "overactive" in some ways but ineffective in others
    - Recurrent sinus infections, bronchitis, UTIs, viral reactivations such as Epstein-Barr Virus, chronic bacterial infections such as Lyme disease, and coinfections

4. Mitochondrial Dysfunction
    - Cytokine storm and oxidative stress impair mitochondrial function and energy production (think Covid)
    - Leads to chronic fatigue, muscle weakness, post-exertional malaise

5. Neuroinflammation
    - Brain fog, memory loss, difficulty concentrating
    - Sleep disturbance, mood swings, depression, anxiety
    - Neuropathic pain or "burning" sensations
    - Long-term risk: cognitive decline and neurodegeneration

6. Hormonal Dysregulation
    - Suppression of hypothalamic-pituitary-adrenal-gonadal axis
    - Low cortisol output (when it becomes chronic)
    - Sex hormone imbalances (low testosterone, menstrual irregularities, LH/FSH ratio elevation such as with PCOS)
    - Thyroid dysfunction (central or as with Hashimoto's—autoimmune)

7. Vascular and Circulatory Problems
    - Endothelial dysfunction (impaired nitric oxide signaling)
    - Reduced oxygen delivery—shortness of breath, exercise intolerance, cold extremities
    - Capillary hypoperfusion (brain and other organs not getting enough blood flow)

8. Detoxification Impairments
    - Downregulation of detox genes (such as glutathione pathways)
    - Chemical sensitivity, poor tolerance of medications or supplements
    - Accumulation of biotoxins and heavy metals

9. Allergy/Mast Cell Activation
    - Mast cell activation syndrome (MCAS): flushing, hives, GI upset, headaches
    - Heightened food sensitivities and histamine tolerance
10. Systemic Multi-Organ Effects
    - GI tract: IBS, bloating, dysbiosis, leaky gut
    - Skin: rashes, eczema, psoriasis
    - Musculoskeletal: chronic pain, fibromyalgia-like symptoms
    - Kidney/Liver: impaired detox and filtering capacity

In autoimmune disease, the immune system loses its delicate balance. When exposed to certain triggers, the regulatory side of immunity—the TH1 helper cells that act like steering wheel and brakes—loses control. Meanwhile, the TH2 side becomes overactive and gets stuck in a heightened state. This creates an unchecked imbalance that affects not just the immune system broadly, but also the gut lining specifically, allowing the overactive immune response to go awry.

I mentioned Hashimoto's thyroiditis earlier in the book, and it perfectly illustrates this process as well. The immune system commonly produces antibodies against gluten proteins. However, some thyroid gland proteins look remarkably similar to gluten proteins from the immune system's perspective. This similarity triggers a case of mistaken identity—the antibodies designed to target gluten begin attacking thyroid tissue instead. This molecular mimicry initiates the autoimmune cascade where our immune system erroneously destroys our own tissue.

The same mechanism applies to virtually all autoimmune diseases. In rheumatoid arthritis, evidence suggests that the immune system creates complexes against specific mycoplasma bacteria, attacking bacteria and the surrounding joint tissue simultaneously.

Even degenerative disc disease follows this pattern, and scientists have found the same bacteria responsible for acne within spinal discs. This raises a fascinating question: Is the problem an overactive immune system attacking these bacteria and disc tissue, or is it an *underactive* immune system that allows these microbes to migrate into tissues where they don't belong?

This dual perspective highlights the complexity of autoimmune disease—it's not simply about immune hyperactivity, but rather a fundamental dysregulation that can manifest as both excessive and insufficient immune responses.

The Importance of Sleep

A good night's sleep carries profound implications on our immune systems. Sleep impacts how these systems function in subduing chronic inflammation, healing injury, fending off disease, and many other scenarios. Moreover, consistent sleep strengthens the immune system, allowing for balanced and effective immune function.[20] We also know that not enough sleep wears down the body's ability to maintain its optimal operation and has great propensity to make you sick.

In my practice, patients with chronic inflammatory response syndrome reveal profound immune dysfunction directly linked to inadequate sleep. These individuals consistently demonstrate suboptimal natural killer (NK) cell activity—a critical finding since NK cells serve as the immune system's first line of defense against infections, tumor cells, and developing cancers.

Of important note is that sleep deprivation almost always creates a cascade of immune deficiencies that extends far beyond NK cells. T-cell function becomes significantly compromised, disrupting what immunologists call cell-mediated immunity. This is particularly concerning because T-cells are essential for fighting infections, coordinating immune responses, and maintaining immunological memory. When T-cell function declines, the body loses its ability to mount effective defenses against pathogens it has previously encountered.

Disrupted antibody production and immune signaling are also of importance. Adequate sleep is fundamental for antibody production—the specialized proteins that target and neutralize specific pathogens. Without sufficient restorative sleep, the body cannot manufacture these targeted immune weapons effectively, leaving individuals vulnerable to infections they should normally resist.

Sleep deprivation also disrupts cytokine production, the crucial signaling molecules that orchestrate immune responses. These chemical messengers coordinate communication between different immune cells, regulate inflammation, and determine the intensity and duration of immune responses. When cytokine production becomes dysregulated due to sleep loss, the entire immune network loses its ability to respond appropriately to threats.

> **Adequate sleep is fundamental for antibody production that targets and neutralizes specific pathogens.**

You can also look at it in terms of mitochondrial function. Lack of quality sleep is extremely detrimental to our mitochondria. Without proper restorative sleep, the mitochondria become fragmented, inefficient, oxidatively stressed, and unable to produce ATP, optimally setting the stage for immune dysfunction, inflammation/inflammaging, chronic fatigue, and so on.

It's a vicious cycle, to say the least. Sleep deprivation affects immune health from multiple angles simultaneously. In individuals with pre-existing immune imbalances, chronic sleep loss exacerbates existing dysfunction, creating a downward spiral of worsening immune competence. The already compromised immune system becomes increasingly unable to perform its protective functions.

More alarmingly, when sleep deprivation extends beyond a few isolated nights and becomes chronic, it can actually trigger immune imbalance in previously healthy individuals. This creates a self-perpetuating cycle: Poor sleep disrupts immune function, which can lead to increased susceptibility to infections and inflammatory conditions, which in turn further disrupts sleep quality. Once this cycle begins, it tends to snowball, with each component reinforcing the others in a progressively worsening pattern of immune dysfunction and sleep disruption.

Emotional and Social Well-Being

Outside the body, positive relationships, support networks, and a sense of belonging can strengthen immune function, while loneliness, stress, and social isolation can increase susceptibility to illness.

For example, research has shown that anxious thoughts can measurably suppress immune response within just thirty minutes—a finding that underscores how intimately our mental and physical health are intertwined. When stress becomes persistent rather than acute, it inflicts lasting damage on the body's natural defense mechanisms, creating vulnerability to infections and chronic illness that might otherwise be easily resisted.

This emotional-immune connection works both ways. Meaningful social interactions serve as powerful immune modulators, actively reducing stress responses while promoting robust immune function. The quality of our relationships and social connections becomes a form of immune medicine, providing protection that extends far beyond emotional comfort.

Every emotion we experience triggers immediate, measurable changes in immune system activity. The immune system doesn't simply observe our emotional states; it actively participates in them. When we laugh, the number and function of immune cells circulating throughout the body change instantly. This is an immediate biological shift that reflects the profound integration between our emotional and immune systems.

Similarly, emotions like crying and anger prompt their own distinct immune responses—whole-body events that reshape our biological state in real time, where the immune system acts as a responder to and participant in our emotional lives:

- Positive emotions such as happiness and joy trigger cascades of beneficial biochemical changes that stimulate the release of endorphins—natural compounds that function as both mood elevators and immune enhancers. Endorphins actively reduce systemic inflammation and promote more balanced, effective immune responses. This creates a positive feedback loop where feeling good literally helps us stay healthy.

- Conversely, negative emotions like sadness and anger activate stress hormone pathways, particularly triggering cortisol release (unless they are already chronically underproducing cortisol). For those who are not underproducing it, elevated cortisol levels create a double burden: they directly suppress immune function while simultaneously promoting inflammatory processes. This combination weakens the body's ability to fight infections and increases susceptibility to inflammatory conditions.[21]

This research reveals that emotional well-being is by no means separate from physical health—it's a core component of immune system maintenance. Our feelings directly influence our body's ability to protect itself, making emotional regulation not just a psychological skill but a crucial aspect of immune health management.

But what happens when it doesn't work out that way? Stress in particular creates a fascinating paradox in immune system behavior. Acute stress—sudden, short-lived challenges that are inevitable in human life—can actually enhance immune function, allowing our bodies to mobilize resources quickly when facing immediate threats, temporarily boosting our ability to fight infections and heal injuries.

However, this beneficial effect only occurs when stress remains acute and brief. The critical distinction lies in chronicity. When stress becomes persistent, it fundamentally alters immune system balance in destructive ways. Chronic stress dysregulates the delicate equilibrium between different immune responses, creating a state of persistent low-grade inflammation that compromises overall immune competence.

Once this immune imbalance establishes itself, it creates a self-perpetuating cycle. Chronic inflammation not only reflects immune dysfunction—it actively worsens it. The inflammatory state disrupts normal immune regulation, making the system increasingly reactive to minor triggers while simultaneously reducing its effectiveness against genuine threats. This progression transforms manageable stress into a significant health liability.

Here's a fascinating exemplar: Many people experience a puzzling pattern of remaining healthy during intensely stressful periods, only to fall ill during vacations or breaks when stress finally subsides. This counterintuitive phenomenon reflects how chronic stress can mask underlying immune dysfunction. During high-stress periods, stress hormones suppress certain immune responses while maintaining others. When stress suddenly decreases, this artificial suppression lifts, often revealing an immune system operating on borrowed time.

Additionally, when people finally relax and "let their guard down," they may encounter new environments, change their routines, or reduce the hypervigilant behaviors that helped them avoid pathogens during stressful periods. The combination of revealed immune dysfunction and increased exposure often results in illness precisely when people expect to feel their best.

The Profound Impact of Social and Emotional Connection

I've seen it time and again in my career, and research consistently demonstrates it—social relationships function as powerful modulators of immune health and overall longevity. Individuals in happy marriages or fulfilling relationships don't just report better quality of life—they actually live longer and maintain stronger immune function throughout their lives. These social connections provide psychological resources that buffer against stress while promoting behaviors and biological processes that support immune health. Broader, strong social support networks can also buffer against stress and improve mental health, positively influencing immune function to promote a healthy immune response.[22]

The mechanisms behind this effect are multifaceted. Positive social relationships reduce chronic stress, promote better sleep, encourage healthier lifestyle choices, and provide emotional support during challenging times. They also appear to directly influence immune function through complex neuroendocrine pathways that researchers are still working to fully understand.

Conversely, loneliness and social isolation create significant health risks that extend far beyond emotional distress. Socially isolated individuals show increased susceptibility to chronic illnesses, accelerated aging processes, and compromised immune responses. The absence of meaningful social connections triggers chronic stress responses similar to those seen with other persistent stressors. When individuals lack social connections, do not practice gratitude, or fail to maintain positive perspectives, they miss crucial protective factors for both immune and mental health. The interconnection between emotional well-being and physical health becomes particularly evident in how psychological states influence everything from infection susceptibility to chronic disease risk.

True health requires a holistic approach that honors the interconnected nature of our body systems.

As a takeaway for this chapter's immune system conversation, we see that true health requires a holistic approach that honors the interconnected nature of our body systems. Quality sleep, balanced exercise, and thoughtful nutrition work synergistically to support immune function and overall vitality. By nourishing our gut microbiome with diverse plant fibers, consuming appropriate amounts of protein, and following seasonal eating patterns, we can create a foundation for lasting health that aligns with both modern science and ancient wisdom.

CHAPTER 7

Brain and Central Nervous System Health

The human brain has 100 billion neurons, each neuron connected to 10,000 other neurons. Sitting on your shoulders is the most complicated object in the universe.

Michio Kaku

The brain is your body's master control center, orchestrating virtually every aspect of human health and function. It regulates movement, immune function, hormones, circadian rhythms, and the biological clock that governs our daily cycles. It also manages our emotions and psychological well-being while simultaneously controlling vital functions such as breathing, heart rate, and digestion.

When brain function is optimized, it creates a cascade of positive effects throughout the entire organism. Conversely, when brain health is compromised, the ripple effects can manifest in seemingly unrelated symptoms across multiple body systems.

So, how do you optimize your brain for peak performance, providing it with the fuel it needs to continuously perform at its highest potential to ensure longevity, cognitive function, and overall well-being? From a big-picture perspective, optimizing brain health requires focusing on the gut-immune system connection, as this profoundly influences brain function. It's a holistic approach that challenges the common tendency to compartmentalize brain health into isolated interventions.

For example, while cognitive exercises like word puzzles have their merit, brain health involves far more complexity than simply "exercising" the brain.

The Gut-Immune System Connection

Multiple interconnected variables contribute to optimal neurological function, making a comprehensive approach—one that includes nutrition, the gut-brain axis, and sleep—essential. Let's tackle each of those one by one.

Nutrition

The therapeutic potential of diet extends back to the 1920s,[23] when researchers discovered that children with epilepsy experienced significant seizure reduction when placed on strict ketogenic diets. This finding revealed how dietary changes and ketone production could stabilize brain function.

The ketogenic diet's effectiveness stems from its ability to enhance mitochondrial function—both improving existing mitochondria and increasing their numbers. This mitochondrial optimization has significant implications for brain stability, raising seizure thresholds and reducing epileptic episodes. Similar stabilizing effects have been observed with omega fatty acids in both epilepsy and bipolar disorder. The brain only accounts for 2 percent of the body's weight, yet it accounts for 20 percent of our ATP production. It is a very metabolically active organ. Because of that, when we improve mitochondrial function, it is typically recognized by improved focus, speed of processing, improved mood stability, and more.

Omega-3 fatty acids represent one of the most well-researched nutrients for brain health. Decades of studies have demonstrated that high-dose omega-3 supplementation can help stabilize conditions like bipolar disorder and seizure disorders, highlighting the profound impact of targeted nutrition on neurological function. Other foundational fats for brain/neurologic health are phospholipids such as phosphotidylcholine, phosphotidylserine, and phosphotidylethanolamine, which become integrated into the lipid bilayer of brain cells. These incredibly important fats can be found in foods such as eggs yolks, liver, meats, fish, shellfish, and certain seeds. A rich supplement source is organic sunflower lecithin. Essential omega fatty acids and phospholipids work hand in hand—they are a dynamic duo for the central nervous system (CNS). They support brain structure, signaling, and resilience. Together they maximize resilience, cognition, and neuroprotection. (*See Fig. 3.*)

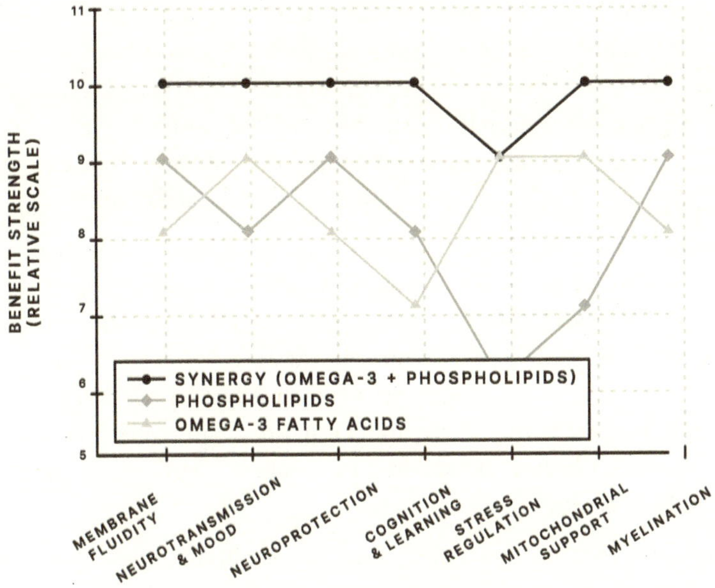

Figure 3. CNS benefits.

Gut-Brain Axis

Let's turn to the gut-brain connection for further insight. The connection between digestive health and brain function extends to fascinating areas like natural hormone production. Research shows that certain fiber blends nourish gut microbiota, increasing bacterial diversity and promoting the growth of specific bacteria that produce our body's own GLP-1 hormones.

These naturally produced GLP-1s function similarly to popular medications like Ozempic and Mounjaro, affecting the brain to suppress appetite and reduce inflammation, demonstrating how proper gut nutrition can naturally replicate pharmaceutical effects through optimized bacterial populations.

Sleep

Sleep enters the picture yet again, representing another fundamental pillar of brain health. Considering that we spend about one-third of our time asleep, quality sleep—and enough of it at the right times—is as essential to survival as food and water. Without sleep, you can't form or maintain the pathways in your brain that allow learning, and a lack of sleep makes it harder to concentrate and to respond quickly. On top of all that, sleep is important to a number of brain functions, including how nerve cells (neurons) communicate with each other.[24]

Understanding the brain's relationships and functions empowers us to make informed decisions about our wellness.

Optimizing brain health truly involves everything. The interconnected nature of nutrition, sleep, gut health, and mitochondrial function creates a complex but manageable system. When we recognize these connections, we can develop more effective, comprehensive strategies for supporting brain health rather than relying on isolated interventions.

The sheer volume and intricacies of the brain's functions are, er, mind-boggling, but understanding these relationships empowers us to make more informed decisions about our overall neurological wellness.

Hormone Dysregulation

One of the most common patterns we see in people with chronic inflammation is hormone dysregulation. The interconnected nature of inflammation and hormone production creates progressive effects that can significantly impact quality of life—but the good news is that these patterns are measurable and reversible.

Take, for example, the pituitary gland, which produces numerous hormones, including antidiuretic hormone (ADH), a crucial component in water regulation. It's very common in people who have chronic inflammatory response syndrome to find that their antidiuretic hormone levels are extremely low—often unmeasurable, in fact, registering as less than 0.8.

When the body doesn't produce adequate ADH, the kidneys don't receive the proper signal to hold onto water. Instead, water passes right through the system, leading to a frustrating cycle of symptoms: frequent urination, increased thirst, and chronic dehydration. People with this condition pee a lot, drink a lot, and are never properly hydrated despite constant fluid intake.

Case Study: Chronic Inflammatory Response Syndrome

PATIENT PROFILE

Age/Sex: 22-year-old male

Chief Complaint: Brain fog and memory lapses

History of Present Illness: Recently returned from a two-year proselytizing mission in Central America. During his service, he developed significant anxiety, insomnia, worsening fatigue, and severe brain fog associated with memory lapses. These symptoms progressed to depression, for which he was prescribed antipsychotic medications. The medications contributed to rapid weight gain and prediabetes.

FUNCTIONAL MEDICINE WORKUP

A comprehensive evaluation revealed evidence of chronic inflammatory response syndrome (CIRS) as the underlying driver of his illness. Key findings included:

- Endocrine/Immune: Hashimoto's thyroiditis with overt hypothyroidism
- Laboratory Abnormalities
  - Elevated Transforming Growth Factor Beta-1 (TGF-β1)
  - Unmeasurable melanocyte-stimulating hormone (MSH)
  - Elevated Matrix Metalloproteinase-9 (MMP-9)
  - Positive thyroid peroxidase antibodies

- Metabolic
- BMI increased from 24 (baseline) to 32 after five months on antipsychotics
    - Hemoglobin A1c: 6.1
    - Fasting leptin: 35

FUNCTIONAL MEDICINE INTERVENTIONS

A targeted, root-cause approach was implemented:

- Diet: Strict gluten-free, anti-inflammatory diet
- Foundational Supplements: Omega-3 fatty acids, phospholipid supplementation, liposomal curcumin
- Immune/Inflammatory Modulation:
    - Low-dose naltrexone
    - Thymogen Alpha-1 and TB4 Frag
    - KPV for low MSH
- Gut Restoration: BPC-157, spore-based probiotics, tributyrin supplementation

OUTCOMES

After eight months of consistent, dedicated adherence:

- Brain fog and memory lapses fully resolved
- Anxiety and depression lifted
- Energy and vitality restored
- Hashimoto's markers improved with thyroid stabilization
- BMI, leptin, and glycemic markers trended toward normalization
- Successfully reintegrated into a university setting, thriving academically and socially with a positive outlook

SUMMARY

This case highlights how a precision functional medicine approach, addressing immune dysregulation, thyroid autoimmunity, metabolic imbalance, and gut dysfunction, can restore cognitive performance, mood stability, and metabolic health—even after severe CIRS-related decline.

In my practice, we treat CIRS with foundational supplements, restorative sleep, lifestyle changes, and the strategic addition of peptides. In doing so, we consistently see hormone production normalize after four to six months. In fact, the day after writing this chapter, I saw three patients whose ADH levels went from unmeasurable (less than 0.8) to normal ranges, and their associated symptoms had completely resolved.

Another critical example involves melanocyte-stimulating hormone, sometimes called alpha melanocyte-stimulating hormone. This hormone is commonly underproduced in people with CIRS, yet it serves vital functions: regulating the immune system, decreasing inflammation, facilitating healing, and providing significant antimicrobial properties.

Here's where it gets interesting—and we'll explore this more later—when melanocyte-stimulating hormone is low, there is typically an associated overgrowth of a particular staph bacteria called MARCONS (multiple antibiotic resistant coagulase negative staph), which itself produces toxins that dysregulate the pituitary's ability to produce alpha melanocyte-stimulating hormone properly, creating a self-perpetuating cycle. Essentially, this "bad booger" has discovered how to allow it to "thrive" through this mechanism of dysregulation. Fortunately, we have effective ways of treating it and restoring melanocyte-stimulating hormone production to optimal levels.

As we implement comprehensive treatment addressing inflammation, gut health, immune health, neurologic and mitochondrial health, and adding targeted peptides, we consistently see this hormone production normalize, breaking the cycle and restoring proper immune function.

Less frequently, but still significantly, we see disrupted communication between the hypothalamus, pituitary, and adrenal glands regarding cortisol production. When these glands aren't sending proper signals to produce adequate cortisol (one of the body's primary natural anti-inflammatory compounds), patients experience significant fatigue and inflammation. In that scenario, things go from bad to worse.

One of my patients had severely low ACTH (adrenalcorticotropin hormone) and morning cortisol levels. After four to five months of treatment, everything normalized: her ACTH reached normal levels, and her morning cortisol jumped from 6 to 14. (I like to see cortisol levels at 12 or better.) The transformation was remarkable—she now has energy in the morning, experiences less inflammation, and reports significantly reduced generalized musculoskeletal pain.

These examples represent just a few of the pituitary hormones that become dysregulated. What makes this particularly exciting is that we can measure these levels and track their normalization throughout treatment. Documenting these improvements provides both clinical validation and hope for patients who have often struggled with these symptoms for years.

Neuroplasticity

For decades, we accepted the conventional wisdom that brain decline was an inevitable part of aging—once we reached adulthood, our neurons were fixed in number and function, steadily deteriorating with each passing year. This perspective painted a grim picture of memory lapses, slower processing, and cognitive decline as simply the price we paid for growing older.

But groundbreaking research has revealed one of the most extraordinary discoveries in modern neuroscience: neuroplasticity. This is the brain's extraordinary ability to rewire itself, form new connections, and even generate new neurons throughout your lifetime, adapting, learning, and growing stronger even in your seventies, eighties, and beyond.

The brain has an extraordinary ability to rewire itself, form new connections, and even generate new neurons throughout our lifetimes.

Neuroplasticity represents nothing short of a revolution in how we understand brain aging. Rather than viewing cognitive decline as inevitable, we can now approach brain health with the same intentionality we bring to physical fitness. Just as your muscles can grow stronger with the right training at any age, your brain can develop new pathways, recover from injury, and maintain—even enhance—cognitive function.

I participated in a transformative training program in this arena through the Institute for Functional Medicine, hosted by Dr. Dale Bredesen, author of *The End of Alzheimer's.*[25] Among the many case studies he presented, one story stood out with stunning clarity—it could actually measure the brain changing.

The patient was a retired internal medicine physician facing cognitive decline. Using advanced volumetric MRI technology, Dr. Bredesen's team measured the volume of his hippocampus—the brain region critical for memory formation and one of the first areas affected by Alzheimer's disease. The baseline results were sobering: His hippocampal volume registered in the 16th or 17th percentile, meaning his brain had already experienced significant shrinkage.

After nine months of Dr. Bredesen's comprehensive treatment protocol—an approach remarkably similar to what I now use in treating chronic inflammatory conditions—they repeated the volumetric MRI. The results defied conventional expectations: The patient's hippocampal volume had jumped to the 76th percentile.

In less than a year, this physician's brain had not only stopped shrinking—it had measurably grown. The hippocampus had regenerated tissue, rebuilt connections, and restored function to levels well above average for his age group.

More than just improvement in symptoms or test scores, this was visible, measurable proof of neuroplasticity in action—the brain's remarkable ability to rebuild, rewire, and regenerate itself. Modern volumetric MRI technology now allows us to witness what was once considered impossible: an aging brain literally growing stronger.

What if we could harness this proven capacity for neuroplasticity before decline sets in? It wasn't long ago when I was in medical school, and we were essentially taught that the brain could not regenerate. But today's research proves it can. Now let's explore how to make it practical.

Strategies for Enhancing Brain Health

There are all kinds of different, interconnected variables that can affect brain health. My approach is to hit it from every angle we can so that we can optimize our brain and overall health.

Exercise

Let's start with exercise. If your brain possesses this extraordinary capacity for renewal, why aren't you thinking about brain fitness the same way you think about physical fitness? We don't think twice about hitting the gym or running a 5k or doing a dedicated yoga routine, but how often do you consider what you could do to make your brain stronger? The truth is, most of us walk around every day without giving a second thought to brain health—until something goes wrong.

When we exercise, we're deliberately hurting ourselves—causing controlled stress that forces our body to adapt and grow stronger. Most people understand this concept when it comes to building muscle or improving cardiovascular health. But what many don't realize is that this same principle of beneficial stress creates some of the most profound changes in your brain.

Recent studies have suggested that the parts of the brain that control thinking and memory are larger in volume in people who exercise than in people who don't. One finding suggests that engaging in a program of regular exercise of moderate intensity over six months or a year is associated with an increase in the volume of selected brain regions.[26]

Consider this: When you engage in high-intensity exercise, especially in a fasted state, you're not just challenging your muscles—you're stressing your mitochondria, the cellular powerhouses that fuel every function in your body. These microscopic engines respond to that stress in remarkable ways: they improve their efficiency, multiply in number, and enhance their performance. This mitochondrial transformation doesn't just affect your physical stamina—it directly impacts your brain in ways that are both measurable and life-changing.

The brain is extraordinarily metabolically active, consuming a disproportionate amount of your body's energy resources. This makes it particularly sensitive to mitochondrial health. As researcher Dr. Chris Palmer, M.D. from Harvard demonstrates in his groundbreaking work *Brain Energy*,[27] metabolic health directly correlates with brain health—whether we're talking about mood, focus, dementia, or cognitive decline. As we improve our metabolic health through mitochondrial optimization, the brain follows suit.

But the exercise-brain connection operates through multiple pathways. When you push your body through challenging exercise, you trigger the production of endorphins—your body's natural response to self-imposed stress. These endorphins don't just improve mood and reduce cravings; they serve as powerful immune modulators, helping to balance an overactive immune system and reduce the chronic inflammation that threatens brain health.

The research clearly identifies how exercise significantly boosts brain health by improving memory, enhancing cognitive function, and reducing the risk of dementia. It promotes neurogenesis—the growth of new brain cells—while enhancing the connections between them.

Nutrition

Yet exercise represents just one piece of the brain health puzzle. The foods you eat—particularly omega-3 fatty acids from sources like fatty fish, antioxidants from berries and leafy greens, phospholipids (from lecithin supplementally), and essential vitamins like B-vitamins, vitamin D, magnesium, and more—all contribute through their own sophisticated mechanisms.

Take omega-3s, for example. These essential fatty acids become incorporated into cell membranes throughout your brain, improving membrane fluidity and functionality. Meanwhile, the ubiquitous seed oils in our modern diet do exactly the opposite—making membranes rigid, promoting inflammation, and causing mitochondrial dysfunction.

The brain, being such a fatty organ, is particularly vulnerable to these membrane changes. When we optimize these foundational elements—exercise, nutrition, and metabolic health—we're not just preventing decline. We're actively building a more resilient, efficient, and capable brain.

Cognitive Function

This begs an interesting question. If you're training for a marathon, dedicated to building muscle mass, or pushing toward a Pacific Crest Trail thru-hike, visible benchmarks allow you to see progress in real time. Your marathon training blocks get faster, your biceps get bigger, you start notching 20-mile trail days. But how do you know if your brain is getting stronger?

There's no easy way to objectively measure cognitive improvement, but most people can recognize it when it happens. A lot of the patients I see who suffer with chronic inflammatory response syndrome have what they call brain fog. While it's subjective, the improvement is very noticeable when that brain fog lifts. We see this all the time as people go through treatment protocols.

One related supplement that is particularly interesting is methylene blue. It was developed in the late 1800s as a textile dye, and they discovered its health benefits almost by accident. During malaria outbreaks, people working in factories that used this textile dye were much less likely to develop malaria symptoms. Interestingly, the drug hydroxychloroquine was actually developed from methylene blue.

Here's the strange part: Methylene blue turns your urine blue but has a very significant impact on mitochondrial health. Most people, especially those suffering with brain fog, notice improvements within a very short period of time when they start taking it as a supplement, experiencing increased focus, improved cognition and clarity, and better processing speed. Most of the time they also notice improvement in overall energy and well-being.

If someone's cognition is already optimal, they probably won't notice much difference, but most of the patients I see suffer with some degree of cognitive brain fog, and they respond nicely to these treatments.

The Power of Restorative Sleep

We've talked about sleep a great deal in these chapters already, and I can't stress it enough. Restorative sleep is wildly powerful in augmenting overall well-being and your best health. From a supplement perspective, some of the peptides we use are phenomenal for boosting brain health, including Epitalon, which significantly improves deep and REM sleep. It doesn't take long for patients to recognize improvements in cognition and focus, especially if they haven't previously been getting proper restorative sleep. Once they start sleeping well, they can really see and feel the difference. As a side note, this marvelous peptide also lengthens telomeres, significantly extending lifespan.

Now, if your body is rested and your brain is already functioning well—if you've got the diet dialed in, the exercise routine, everything optimized for your brain and physical health—then it's more preemptive. You can't look inside your brain and say, "Hey, look, it's getting stronger," but you know you're doing the right things.

Restorative sleep is a powerful component in augmenting overall well-being and your best health.

That being said, we should turn our attention to omega-3s again, which support everything from brain structure and function to mood and cognitive performance. DHA, one of the key components in fish oil, is a crucial structural component of brain cells. It integrates into the brain's structure and helps maintain the fluidity and integrity of nerve cell membranes, which are essential for proper neuron function.

Neurons are long, streamy cells that are primarily composed of membranes. When omega-3s get integrated into the cell structure, they drastically improve functionality. We've also seen that higher omega-3 levels are associated with larger hippocampal volumes, a significant point, as the hippocampus is the brain region that tends to shrink in Alzheimer's disease, and it's crucial for all brain function.

While we know that the brain simply does not function well when deprived of restorative sleep, there's one critical aspect we don't think about much that's worth mentioning: brain waste removal.

During sleep, the brain engages in what we call glymphatic flow, which clears waste and toxins from the brain. This is our restorative baseline. Without that glymphatic flow, without ridding the body of those toxins and waste products, they accumulate and have an adverse effect on brain function. Inflammation sets in and worsens when we can't get rid of those brain waste products.

Sleep also protects the brain in very significant ways, including regulating levels of certain proteins that can contribute to degenerative diseases such as Alzheimer's and Parkinson's. For example, as we age—and brain aging is accelerated with chronic inflammation—we may experience pineal gland calcification. In fact, the pineal gland can start to calcify and reduce function as early as age thirty.

Fortunately, there's a lot we can do to help restore that function. The peptide Epitalon, mentioned previously, can actually reset and, to some degree, regrow the pineal gland, helping it function better. Since the pineal gland controls our circadian rhythms (and our biological clock), when we reset it, we can see significant enhancement in both the quality and quantity of restorative sleep. This has a tremendous impact on brain health, neuroplasticity, and the brain's ability to rid itself of accumulated toxins.

So, does good sleep clear out mental waste—your overload of thoughts and emotional baggage? That's harder to measure, but it's absolutely true. Our emotional and mental health are directly proportional to our overall brain health. If the brain is inflamed because we're not getting rid of toxins, or because the gut isn't healthy, the microbiome is off, or the immune system is compromised—all those things negatively impact the brain, mood, and emotions.

Sleep has a significant emotional impact. People who are sleep deprived simply don't tend to be happy, try as they may. Having a positive mental attitude is key, even when we're struggling through trials, but sleep is critical for that emotional component.

Everything plays off each other. If I go to bed stressed about something or with a million things on my mind, I can't sleep. But if there are toxins in my brain or other issues preventing good sleep, then I don't sleep because of that either. It all tends to spiral.

Unfortunately, modern medicine wants to prescribe us sleep medications, though study after study shows these are bad for the brain. Ambien (zolpidem), for example, has been shown to adversely affect memory. People easily get caught in this cycle where they're desperate for sleep, which worsens their emotional health and perpetuates insomnia.

When we intervene with prescription sleep medications, we don't address the root cause, and we don't improve our mental or emotional health; quite the contrary. These drugs, with continued use, worsen anxiety, memory, cognition, and depression. You can also experience rebound anxiety when the medication wears off.

Even melatonin, which seems so innocent, isn't something you want to take every night. That's because doing so can cause you to produce less of your own natural melatonin. The pineal gland produces the body's melatonin, so when we reset that gland, we start producing melatonin properly on our own. There's no downside to that.

All told, melatonin can be problematic, especially at higher doses, as it can potentially cause rebound insomnia and can reduce our natural production. It's certainly less concerning than prescription sleep medications, but it's not a great long-term solution.

Emotional Health and the Mind-Body Connection

Emotional health plays a significant role in brain health. We are beings made of highly intricate, interconnected components, and emotional well-being has a direct, measurable impact on brain function and structure.

When I see patients struggling with chronic stress, unresolved trauma, or persistent anxiety, I consistently observe corresponding issues with cognitive function. It's not just that they "feel bad," their brains are literally functioning differently. Chronic emotional stress triggers inflammatory cascades that directly affect neural pathways, memory formation, and executive function. The hippocampus, that critical area for learning and memory that we mentioned earlier, actually shrinks under prolonged emotional stress.

Emotional well-being has a direct, measurable impact on brain health.

But emotional distress isn't just "in your head," it creates real, physical changes in brain tissue. Chronic stress opens the door for chronic inflammation, which, over time, damages brain cells and disrupts the delicate balance of neurotransmitters. This is why patients with untreated depression or anxiety often struggle with brain fog, memory issues, and difficulty concentrating. Their emotional state is literally impairing their cognitive machinery. It becomes a vicious cycle.

However, the brain has remarkable plasticity. When we address emotional health through proper therapy, emotional awareness, and healthy coping mechanisms, we see corresponding improvements in brain function. I've watched patients' cognitive clarity return as they work through emotional trauma or learn more comprehensive, effective stress management techniques.

And therapy is good brain medicine. Whether it's cognitive behavioral therapy, EMDR for trauma, or even simple mindfulness practices, these interventions create measurable changes in brain structure and function. A resulting emotional awareness—learning to recognize and process feelings rather than suppressing them—literally rewires neural pathways in beneficial ways.

Healthy coping mechanisms are equally crucial. I've seen patients transform their cognitive function by developing better emotional regulation skills. Simple practices like breathing exercises, meditation, journaling, or even regular physical exercise don't just improve mood; they preserve and enhance brain health over time.

In the long run, patients who do best are those who understand that emotional health isn't separate from physical health. When someone learns to process grief, to forgive, to be grateful, to manage anxiety effectively, or break free from chronic stress patterns, their brain function improves dramatically. Taking care of your emotional well-being is one of the most powerful things you can do for your brain health, and the effects compound over time.

Now, all of this brain optimization—sleep, omega-3 and phospholipid-rich foods and/or supplementation, and emotional health—comes down to one fundamental level: the mitochondria. These are the powerhouses of our cells, and when we're talking about brain health, we're really talking about mitochondrial health. Let's dive into why these tiny cellular engines are so critical to everything we've been discussing.

CHAPTER 8

Mitochondrial Health

Mitochondria are not just the powerhouse of the cell; they are the guardians of life and longevity.

Functional Medicine axiom

Sarah's familiar afternoon crash arrived right on schedule. It was just 2 p.m., yet she felt like she'd been awake for days, despite her morning vitamins, carefully planned salad lunch, and motivational podcasts on the way to work. Supplement bottles, lined up like tiny soldiers on her windowsill—B-complex, iron, vitamin D, magnesium—held promises of energy that never quite delivered. Sarah also suffered from chronic fatigue, brain fog, and recurrent sinus infections in addition to her afternoon crashes. History was significant for mold exposure, poor sleep, a processed diet, and hypothyroidism.

Labs showed elevated inflammatory markers, abnormal lactate to pyruvate ratio, low CoQ10 and carnitine levels, oxidative stress, and a flattened cortisol curve—all consistent with mitochondrial dysfunction and chronic inflammation (CIRS).

What is the secret to boundless energy? Is it lots of sleep and vegetables? Extra vitamins? Exercise and a positive attitude? Those things certainly contribute, and I recommend them all. But the big-ticket ingredient is your mitochondria, your body's powerhouse.

Most people have never heard of these microscopic marvels, yet they hold the key to everything we feel and do. Even now, as you read this chapter, trillions of these cellular engines are humming along, converting the food you ate into the energy that drives you. They are literally the reason you can think, move, breathe, and dream. They're also the reason why some mornings you bound out of bed ready to conquer the world, while other days you can barely summon the energy to get out the door.

The difference between feeling vibrant as opposed to drained is more than what you put in your body; it's how efficiently these tiny dynamos can transform it into usable energy. And you are at the controls, as your mitochondria are incredibly trainable, adaptable, and responsive to the choices you make every single day.

So what was our intervention for Sarah? An anti-inflammatory diet, removal of inciting triggers, improved sleep, and replenishment of mitochondrial nutrients, including NAD+ optimization strategies. Then, intermittent fasting, hyperbaric oxygen therapy with red light therapy, hormetic stressors such as heat and cold, progressive exercise, and peptides.

Outcome: Within six months, Sarah reported restored sleep and energy, sharper cognition, improved mood, weight loss, no further sinus infections, improved HRV (heart rate variability), normalization of inflammatory markers and pituitary hormones, and improved mitochondrial markers.

Conclusion: Sarah has her life back, she has her optimal health back, and she is motivated to keep it that way.

This chapter sheds light on why your mitochondria might be running at half-speed, and more importantly, how to unleash their full potential.

Mitochondria in Action

When I educate my patients one-on-one, I like using the analogy that mitochondria recharge our cellular batteries. And if those aren't recharging optimally, our health is going to suffer, and it suffers across the board because we have mitochondria in every single cell (except for mature red blood cells).

To start, let's take a high-level look at mitochondria in action. Properly functioning mitochondria impact energy levels, metabolic processes, and cell longevity. When they're working as they should, our overall health responds in kind. However, disruptions in mitochondrial function can lead to a host of health issues from fatigue and metabolic disorders to neurodegenerative diseases.[28]

Everything from energy production to brain function is at work here. Most of your body's energy is mitochondria generated in the form of ATP—the molecular currency that powers every cellular process. When mitochondrial function falters, persistent fatigue replaces vitality, physical performance diminishes, and organ systems struggle to maintain their essential functions.[29] There's also a direct correlation with mitochondria and aging, as mitochondrial function declines with age. In that regard, if we can optimize mitochondrial health, we can slow the aging process, improve quality of life, and make an enormous difference in our health.

But energy production represents only the beginning of mitochondria's influence on your health and longevity. Beyond their role as cellular powerhouses, mitochondria serve as sophisticated command centers, directing the complex signaling networks that govern cellular behavior. Your cells are programmed to perform specific functions—producing essential proteins, responding to environmental cues, maintaining tissue integrity—but these processes require optimal mitochondrial function to operate at their full potential.

Perhaps most crucially, healthy mitochondria regulate apoptosis—the programmed death of cells that have outlived their usefulness or become damaged. This process isn't destructive; it's essential for renewal and optimal function. When mitochondria lose their capacity to effectively manage cellular turnover, dysfunctional cells accumulate rather than being cleared away.[30] This is termed cellular senescence.

This breakdown in cellular housekeeping accelerates aging and creates an environment where cellular damage compounds over time. The result is a gradual decline in tissue function and an increased vulnerability to age-related diseases.

A breakdown in cellular housekeeping creates an environment of compounding cellular damage.

A Cascade of Systemic Impact

The consequences of mitochondrial dysfunction extend far beyond fatigue or cellular damage. Because the most metabolically active organs—your brain and heart—depend heavily on efficient energy production, mitochondrial impairment often manifests most dramatically in these systems. Neurological and neurodegenerative disorders frequently trace their origins to mitochondrial dysfunction, with their connections extending to mental health conditions including anxiety, depression, bipolar disorder, and various autism spectrum disorders. This relationship underscores the profound connection between cellular energy production and neurological function.[31]

Let's look closer at the mental health element, which plays such an important role in our lives and, if left unattended or damaged, can have lasting, debilitating effects. Mitochondrial and mental health are intricately connected, and dysfunction in the former can drastically impact the latter. Mitochondria play a direct role in generating the energy our brains need to carry out everyday processes, including mood regulation, thinking tasks, and memory. The brain is a very metabolically active organ, and without adequate energy, we feel fatigue, cognitive sluggishness, and difficulty focusing—all common ingredients in various mental health conditions.[32]

In his book *Brain Energy*, Dr. Chris Palmer builds on his comprehensive research in mental health, conducted in his roles at Harvard Medical School and McLean Hospital. Palmer sums it up perfectly: "Mental disorders—all of them—are metabolic disorders of the brain."[33] Palmer's narrative discusses how psychological stress can negatively impact mitochondrial function, leading to a state of mitochondrial allostatic load (chronic stress), and this is what happens with chronic inflammatory response syndrome. It can disrupt mitochondrial metabolism and increase oxidative stress, contributing to the development of worsening mental health issues. This circles back to our earlier discussion of the cell danger response and its association with adverse childhood experiences or early life trauma. Those experiences spark a survival mechanism that adversely affects mitochondrial health and often leads to mental health challenges later in life.

> **"Mental disorders are metabolic disorders of the brain."**
>
> DR. CHRIS PALMER

For example, a friend of mine shared his story of familial trauma that manifested his inner protector to behave a certain way in light of others' expectations and judgement. This essentially reshaped his person for decades, impacting marriage, parenthood, friendships, and career. It wasn't until a therapist introduced the protector element, awareness, and reidentifying with who he wanted to be that he was able to lean in and reset.

Cardiovascular health represents another critical battleground. Your heart muscle requires tremendous energy to maintain its relentless rhythm, making it particularly vulnerable when mitochondrial function declines. The intricate relationship between cellular energy production and cardiac performance explains why mitochondrial support often yields dramatic improvements in cardiovascular health.

Understanding these fundamental relationships becomes the foundation for everything that follows. The most sophisticated supplementation protocols and advanced interventions mean little without grasping why mitochondrial health matters profoundly. When you recognize that these cellular powerhouses influence everything from your daily energy levels to your long-term neurological health, the commitment to optimization becomes essential.

The journey toward extraordinary mitochondrial health—and the vibrant life it enables—begins with this understanding. From here, we can build the comprehensive approach that transforms cellular function and unlocks your body's full potential.

Of course, the road to health is almost always littered with potholes, confusing intersections, and occasional dead ends. For example, immune dysfunction inspires inflammation, which then adversely affects the mitochondria, and then the mitochondria worsen immune function and inflammation, churning in a vicious cycle.

One of my approaches to achieving overall whole health and well-being is to hit it from every angle we possibly can. Unsurprisingly, some of my patients become overwhelmed by the dizzying array of recommendations I give them, but this is the best way to optimize their chance of success.

Many people I work with are metabolically not in a good place because of their diet. To really change mitochondrial health, you have to be willing to go to a strict low-carbohydrate, ketogenic type of diet for its mitochondrial-enhancing impact. That alone can make an enormous difference in mitochondrial health. Now, that doesn't mean turning your meals into a joyless routine. It's okay to earn our dietary indiscretions. If we really buckle down, make goals, and stick to them as best we can, then we start to see those metabolic mitochondrial changes manifest themselves. We become more metabolically flexible. When that happens (when we're a good distance down the mitochondrial enhancement pathway), a few dietary indiscretions from time to time won't set us back or cause harm because we've primed our metabolism to tolerate them without causing damage. Still, a lot of people will dig in their heels and say, "Hold on a minute. Am I going to have to eat this way indefinitely?" The answer is no. It won't be easy, but when you do the work at the outset, you'll realize optimal health faster. Then you can let the pedal off the gas, and an indiscretion from time to time won't matter.

Best of all, after locking in the dietary habits, they naturally become part of your routine, and when you learn to love your new vibrant lifestyle, you'll want to "do what you gotta do" to maintain it.

Mitochondrial Health and Optimization

When you're ready to move beyond basic function to true optimization, supporting your mitochondria is critical. Fueling that function comes in the form of a who's who of powerful essential nutrients.

Omega fatty acids form the foundation of mitochondrial health as well, providing the structural components these organelles need to thrive. Fish oil supplementation offers one pathway, but the real transformation comes through a comprehensive approach that includes targeted nutrients working in synergy.

Alpha lipoic acid stands out as a master antioxidant, protecting your cells directly while regenerating other antioxidants, creating a cascading effect of cellular protection. This compound exemplifies true optimization: one intervention amplifying the benefits of others.

Coenzyme Q10, particularly in its active form ubiquinol, serves as a crucial component in electron transport—the very process that generates ATP. Without adequate CoQ10, your mitochondria simply cannot produce energy efficiently.

L-carnitine works alongside this system, facilitating the transport of fatty acids into the mitochondria where they can be converted to fuel.[34]

The B-Complex vitamins represent another cornerstone of mitochondrial support. These nutrients work collectively in energy production pathways, each playing specific roles that cannot be replicated by others (typically recommended in their methylated/active forms).

Magnesium plays a big role as well, serving as a cofactor in hundreds of enzymatic reactions, many of which are essential for optimal mitochondrial function.

Creatine deserves special recognition beyond traditional supplementation. While most people use it for muscle building, its effects on mitochondrial health extend far beyond the gym. By supporting mitochondrial function, creatine enhances cognitive performance and overall cellular energy production. This connection between physical and mental performance illustrates the integrated nature of true health optimization.

Through it all, the real power lies in understanding how lifestyle factors amplify these nutrients' effects.

The Hormetic Principle

What makes mitochondria stronger mirrors what makes us stronger as individuals: strategic challenge followed by recovery. This principle, known as hormesis, explains why certain interventions that temporarily stress the system ultimately enhance its function.

Here's how it works: A healthy ketogenic diet forces mitochondria to adapt by restricting their preferred fuel source—sugar in the form of glucose. This metabolic challenge, when applied thoughtfully, strengthens mitochondrial function over time. Similarly, intermittent fasting and exercising in a fasted state create adaptive stress that enhances mitochondrial function and cellular resilience. However, keep in mind that this principle has boundaries. For example, while we can strategically restrict certain fuels or challenge our systems through exercise, we cannot compromise restorative sleep and expect positive adaptation. Sleep remains non-negotiable—it's during these hours that mitochondria recover and regenerate.

Other emerging compounds include NAD+ (see below), urolithin A, PQQ, quercetin, apigenin, EGCG, antioxidants that protect the mitochondria (Vitamins C, E, glutathione and its precursors, selenium, zinc, resveratrol, and curcumin), phospholipids, cardiolipin support, taurine, adaptogens, polyphenols, citrulline, Shilajit, astaxanthin, and Vitamin K2 (mk7).

The NAD+ Revolution

Perhaps no area of mitochondrial medicine holds more promise than NAD+ optimization. This crucial coenzyme, essential for energy production and cellular repair, naturally declines with age and chronic inflammation. The ratio of NAD+ to its reduced form, NADH, serves as a key indicator of mitochondrial health.

We can restore NAD+ levels through direct supplementation—intravenous or subcutaneous administration provides rapid results but requires significant time and financial investment (there is emerging evidence that liposomal NAD+ can work in oral form). A more accessible approach involves NAD+ precursors, with niacinamide (vitamin B3) offering an inexpensive yet effective option for most people.

The future may hold even more targeted interventions. Compounds like 5-Amino-1MQ work differently—rather than increasing NAD+ production, they slow its breakdown, supporting the crucial NAD+/NADH ratio from the other direction.

This brings me to an additional thought on "lifestyle supplementation." Regular physical activity is one of the best ways to support mitochondrial health, particularly aerobic and resistance exercise, to increase muscle cell density and boost energy production. This all makes sense in theory, but what does it look like in the real world?

Exercise makes life difficult for mitochondria, and they respond by multiplying. More mitochondria means more energy means reduced risk of related diseases. And one way we can enhance those benefits is to exercise in a fasted or low-carbohydrate state, which promotes the synthesis of new mitochondria and the removal of damaged ones through a process called mitophagy. The exercise doesn't feel as good, but the payoff is bigger.

So is this approach limited to certain age groups, abilities, or frequency? The short answer is that *all* exercise is good for you and critical for overall health. Walking around the block three times a week or crushing a sufferfest HIIT workout will both promote mitochondrial biogenesis in different amounts. Running, swimming, and cycling are arguably the big highly beneficial endurance activities, but whatever your passion, know that exercise works equally as well as, if not better than, antidepressants such as Prozac for treatment of depression,[35] without all the side effects. For this, you can thank your endorphin pathways. During exercise, endorphins immunomodulate (alter the immune system's activity to maintain the body's defense mechanisms), playing a vital role in maintaining homeostasis and contributing to enduring physical health and emotional well-being.

Ultimately, true mitochondrial optimization requires the same level of commitment you'd bring to any meaningful pursuit. Whether you're training for a triathlon or cultivating a garden, the depth of your engagement determines your results. Mitochondrial health is no different—you can maintain basic function, or you can pursue extraordinary cellular vitality. The latter, of course, demands integration across all dimensions of health. Physical protocols without mental commitment produce limited results. Supplementation without lifestyle optimization remains incomplete. Full engagement is required, and the end product speaks for itself.

PART THREE

Treatment—How to Heal and Optimize

You've reached the critical juncture where knowledge transforms into power. The first two parts of this book equipped you with the foundation—understanding how chronic inflammation develops and recognizing its far-reaching impact on every system in your body. Now comes the most important phase: translating that understanding into concrete action that will fundamentally change your health trajectory.

This isn't just adding another supplement to your morning routine or trying the latest health trend for a few weeks before abandoning it. What you're about to embark on represents a comprehensive approach to reclaiming your biological potential. The strategies outlined in this section address the root causes of dysfunction rather than merely managing symptoms because true healing requires us to work upstream from where conventional medicine typically intervenes.

The modern world has created unprecedented challenges for human health, but it has also provided us with unprecedented tools for optimization. We now have access to precision approaches that can target specific pathways, support cellular function at the mitochondrial level, and help your body remember how to regulate inflammation naturally. These aren't experimental treatments—they're evidence-based interventions that address the fundamental mechanisms driving chronic disease.

Your journey toward optimal health will unfold across three strategic levels. First, we'll establish the foundational lifestyle measures that create optimal environmental conditions for healing. These suggestions form the bedrock upon which everything else builds. Without proper sleep architecture, stress management, and movement patterns, even the most advanced therapies will fall short of their potential.

Next, we'll explore targeted nutritional support through foundational supplements that address the nutrient deficiencies and metabolic imbalances that perpetuate inflammatory cycles. This is strategic supplementation in action, based on your individual needs and the specific pathways that require support.

Finally, we'll venture into the cutting-edge realm of peptide therapy, where specific biological messengers can communicate directly with your cells to optimize function, reduce inflammation, enhance recovery, and accelerate healing processes. These powerful tools represent the pinnacle of personalized medicine, allowing us to influence biological processes with remarkable precision.

Throughout this section, you'll notice a consistent theme: empowerment through education and action. Every protocol, every recommendation, every strategy is designed to put you in control of your health outcomes. No longer will you be at the mercy of a system that waits for disease to manifest before taking action. Instead, you'll become the architect of your own vitality.

We begin with a systematic approach to treating chronic inflammation itself. In Chapter 9, you'll learn to identify and eliminate the inflammatory triggers that have been sabotaging your health while implementing targeted interventions that help your immune system remember how to regulate itself properly. This foundation is crucial because without addressing the underlying inflammatory cascade, even the most advanced therapies will struggle to create lasting change.

From there, we'll explore one of the most powerful tools in modern regenerative medicine: peptide therapy. Chapter 10 demystifies these biological messengers that represent a breakthrough in personalized health optimization, capable of communicating directly with your cells to influence healing, recovery, and optimal function. You'll discover how these compounds work, why they're so effective, and how to determine which peptides align with your specific health goals and challenges.

Once you understand both the foundational approach to inflammation and the advanced potential of peptides, Chapter 11 will integrate everything into a comprehensive optimization strategy. This means learning how to layer peptide therapy with strategic supplementation and dietary interventions, creating a personalized protocol that evolves with your changing needs and goals. The key is understanding how these different modalities work synergistically rather than in isolation.

We'll then revisit the critical systems covered in Part Two—gut health, immune function, hormonal balance, detoxification, neurologic and metabolic health—but this time from a treatment perspective. In Chapter 12, you'll discover specific interventions for each system and learn how to address multiple pathways simultaneously for maximum therapeutic benefit. This targeted approach means that no aspect of your health optimization is left to chance.

Chapter 13 ties everything together with a sustainable framework for maintaining your gains and continuing to optimize over time. This is about creating a lifestyle that supports ongoing vitality and resilience, one that adapts as you age and as your circumstances change.

The path ahead requires commitment, but it doesn't require perfection. What it demands is consistency in applying these principles and the willingness to make choices that serve your long-term health rather than short-term convenience. The protocols you're about to learn have the power to reverse years of inflammatory damage and set you on a trajectory toward thriving in health and life.

Your optimal health is a way of being that you can achieve and maintain when you understand how to work with your body's innate healing mechanisms rather than against them. The tools are in your hands.

CHAPTER 9

How to Treat Chronic Inflammation

To treat inflammation is not to silence the immune system, but to restore its balance.

Functional Medicine axiom

Let me start with an example we can all relate to. When you cut your finger, you see redness, swelling, maybe some warmth around the wound. That's acute inflammation, and it's exactly what you want to see. It's your body's natural, necessary response to injury—bringing healing cells to the area, fighting off potential infection, and starting the repair process. This type of inflammation is temporary, targeted, and beneficial.

Chronic inflammation is an entirely different animal. It's like having that same inflammatory response turned on continuously, but without a clear purpose or eventual resolution. Instead of lasting days or weeks to heal a specific injury, chronic inflammation persists for months or years, often without us even realizing it's there.

What makes chronic inflammation so insidious is that it is largely silent. When you see or feel the acute inflammation from that cut on your finger, you know exactly what's happening and where. But chronic inflammation hides in the background, affecting multiple systems in your body simultaneously.

Every thirty-three seconds, someone in America dies from heart disease.[36] Every forty seconds, someone has a stroke.[37] Globally, someone is diagnosed with dementia every 3.2 seconds.[38] You brush your teeth every morning to prevent cavities. You wear sunscreen to avoid skin cancer. You check your blood pressure to help prevent heart disease. But what if the greatest threat to your health is something you can't see or feel, and it could be affecting you right now? What if your body's own healing mechanism has turned traitor while you go about your daily life, with no idea of the invisible threat?

Chronic inflammation is recognized by few but suffered by many. On the path to healing, my approach starts with extensive laboratory analysis, which goes on to specifically guide therapy. But first, we must understand chronic inflammation assessment and treatment.

Acute inflammation is not only expected but is needed and wanted. Normal inflammatory response is necessary for healing. Chronic inflammation, on the flip side, can damage healthy tissues and organs. It's not optimal and has a significant negative impact on our health. That is the primary element we're trying to assess and treat.

People often tell me they've been dealing with brain fog for years, or they just don't have the energy they used to have, or they can't seem to lose weight no matter what they try. They have adapted to feeling this way—it's become their new normal. What they don't realize is that what they're experiencing isn't just "getting older" or stress from work—it's often chronic inflammation quietly damaging their health. Unlike the controlled burn of acute inflammation that clears away damaged tissue and promotes healing, chronic inflammation is like a wildfire, damaging healthy tissues and organs. In the end, what feels like "just getting older" is often a slow-burning inflammatory process beneath the surface.

Chronic inflammation is recognized by few but suffered by many.

At the heart of chronic inflammation is an immune system that's lost balance. Your immune system has two key components (in reality, it is more complex than this, but for discussion purposes, we'll simplify it this way): TH1/TReg and TH2/TH17. The former is targeted, precise, and designed primarily to defend against threats like intracellular viruses and bacteria—considered the cell-mediated immunity (the cytokines interferon-gamma, interleukin-2, and tissue necrosis factor beta). This side (TH1) also enhances NK (natural killer) cell function. The latter, TH2/TH17, is more about defending against extracellular pathogens like parasites and toxins and is considered the more humoral/antibody-driven immunity. This side (TH2) produces the cytokines interleukin-4 (IL-4), IL-5, IL-6, IL-10, and IL-13. It activates B cells, which produce antibodies. It recruits eosinophils, basophils, and mast cells. In chronic inflammation, more often than not, the TH1/TReg side becomes underactive while the TH2/TH17 side becomes overactive, creating inflammation that can go unchecked without the precision targeting/control side (TH1) needed to actually solve the problem. This common imbalance leads to things such as asthma, atopic dermatitis (eczema), food sensitivities, and chronic infections with a weakened ability to clear the infection. Sometimes the TH1 side is overactive, such as with autoimmune flares, whereas the TH2 dominant imbalance invites allergic/inflammatory hypersensitivity and poor clearance of infections (think EBV or chronic Lyme disease, for example). More simply put, TH1 = soldiers with guns (directly attack and kill infected cells) versus TH2 = diplomats and medics (call in antibodies, eosinophils, and mast cells to handle external invaders and toxins). It's a bit confusing, but the take-home point is that we need balance between the two sides, and with chronic inflammation and autoimmune disease, the system is simply dysregulated.

This is where it gets really interesting from a health perspective. Chronic inflammation directly damages your mitochondria. When not properly functioning, this can lead to the persistent fatigue experienced by so many people. It's like your cellular engines are running on half power. That's when things go from bad to worse.

But it goes even deeper. When your mitochondria are damaged, your entire metabolism suffers. When the mitochondria don't make energy efficiently, the cells simply can't do their various jobs effectively. The cells can't meet their energy demands, leading to fatigue, exercise intolerance, and muscle weakness. The higher-energy organs like the brain, heart, liver, kidneys, and muscles are hit the hardest. This low-energy state also leads to more oxidative stress, leading to DNA, protein, and lipid damage (think oxidized LDL cholesterol), triggering more chronic inflammation/inflammaging. This state leads to even more immune dysregulation. It also leads to metabolic dysfunction, including impaired fatty acid oxidation (can't burn fat), leptin and insulin resistance, weight gain, and prediabetes/metabolic syndrome. The mitochondria have become metabolically inflexible (can't switch to fat burning effectively). We also see neurocognitive decline, cellular senescence and accelerated aging, hormonal dysregulation, poor detoxification, and more. Like I said, it goes from bad to far worse!

Left unchecked, chronic inflammation can be a direct route to virtually every major disease we see today:

Heart Disease Risk: Chronic inflammation damages the lining of your arteries, making them more prone to plaque buildup and inflammation in arterial walls. When I see elevated cardio-selective CRP levels, it is an indication of increased heart disease risk.

Diabetes and Metabolic Syndrome: Chronic inflammation also interferes with insulin signaling. Your cells become resistant to insulin, not because they're broken, but because inflammatory signals are blocking the insulin receptors, which can lead to diabetes and metabolic syndrome.

When chronic inflammation persists, your immune system can start attacking your own tissues. This is how we get autoimmune conditions like rheumatoid arthritis, Hashimoto's thyroiditis, and inflammatory bowel disease.

Alzheimer's and Parkinson's Diseases:. On a neurodegenerative level, the brain is particularly vulnerable to chronic inflammation, affecting cognitive function that, over time, can link to conditions like Alzheimer's and Parkinson's disease.

Cancer: Chronic inflammation also creates an environment favorable for cancer development by cultivating a constantly irritated area that's more prone to cellular damage and abnormal growth.

And chronic inflammation doesn't just affect your immune system—it disrupts the entire hormonal operation, inflaming your hypothalamus and pituitary gland to send mixed signals. This is why we see low DHEA sulfate levels, disrupted thyroid function, sex hormone dysregulation, and problems with hormones like ADH and melanocyte-stimulating hormone.

Breaking the Cycle of Chronic Inflammation

As mentioned above, what makes chronic inflammation so challenging is that it damages mitochondria, which reduces your energy production. Low energy means your body can't effectively fight the inflammation. Poor sleep from inflammation makes everything worse. Then we see suboptimal morning cortisol production, which further promotes inflammation. And around and around it goes.

The good news is that chronic inflammation is treatable. Unlike genetic diseases that we can't change, chronic inflammation responds to targeted interventions. When we identify underlying triggers—whether it's gut dysfunction, hormone imbalances, nutritional deficiencies, or toxic exposures—and address them systematically, we can break that cycle.

This goes beyond suppressing inflammation with medications long-term; the key is identifying why your body is inflamed in the first place and fixing those root causes. When we do that, the body's natural healing mechanisms can take over. Fully understanding chronic inflammation gives us a roadmap for getting back to optimal health by restoring the body's natural balance and letting it heal itself.

Of course, the road to healing starts with recognizing symptoms. Chronic inflammation includes a host of indicators, including these top five:

1. **Fatigue** is arguably the most common symptom. In most cases, those suffering with chronic inflammation have mitochondrial dysfunction, which commonly presents as persistent fatigue issues. You'll also experience joint pain or stiffness, muscle aches, and digestive issues.
2. **Gut health** is crucial. There's a very strong connection between gut health and overall inflammation. Interestingly, the gut lining, the skin, and the respiratory tract are the same surface early on in our development (in the embryo). When I see skin problems, I think gut issues in most cases.

3. **Mental and emotional symptoms** are also common: mood issues, depression, anxiety, focus problems, attention issues, and brain fog. Chronic inflammation can certainly affect things metabolically as well, leading to weight problems and other metabolic issues that relate back to mitochondrial dysfunction.
4. **Sleep issues** are another red flag. And if the immune system is weaker than normal, patients may be more susceptible to infections.
5. **Headaches** are another common symptom, along with just not feeling well overall or having a flu-like feeling.

It's important to note that chronic inflammation doesn't necessarily have to present as autoimmune disease, though that can certainly be part of the larger umbrella.

So what is the best approach to address inflammation? "Best" is always the subject of debate, but during initial assessments with patients, I conduct very thorough blood work. Some of these tests are unique to assessing chronic inflammatory response syndrome, but I look very broadly to provide the most promising results.

I start with the fundamentals: complete blood count, metabolic panel, kidney and liver function, and electrolytes. From there, I look thoroughly at hormones, particularly thyroid function. I measure TSH, T3, T4, and reverse T3 and typically include thyroid-associated antibodies such as thyroid peroxidase antibody and thyroidglobulin antibody, which can be associated with Hashimoto's disease and Graves' disease—pretty common autoimmune diseases affecting the thyroid.

I also examine other hormones: female hormones, male hormones, free testosterone, total testosterone, and DHEA sulfate, which is the most abundant hormone in the human body, produced by the adrenal glands. In chronic disease and chronic inflammation, DHEA sulfate production is commonly low. We've been led to believe this is associated with "adrenal fatigue," but the truth is actually broader hormone dysregulation—it's the hypothalamus and pituitary not sending proper signals to the adrenal glands.

Moving on, I look at several key metabolic markers, including measuring hemoglobin A1C, which averages blood sugars over about ninety days, and fasting insulin levels. I also check fasting leptin levels because chronic inflammation very commonly leads to leptin resistance. Leptin is considered the satiety hormone or anti-hunger hormone. When you have leptin resistance, you don't get the hunger shutoff signal like you should, which can lead to weight issues, metabolic problems, insulin resistance, prediabetes, and diabetes.

I also thoroughly examine lipid panels using what's called a lipoprofile NMR (nuclear magnetic resonance—another term for MRI). This technology looks at blood much more accurately by measuring particles in the bloodstream. We can more thoroughly assess lipid and cholesterol levels this way. Traditional cholesterol tests aren't accurately assessing risk, so we use this newer technology for more accurate assessment. It also gives us an insulin resistance score, which is very helpful in determining treatment needs.

On the immune system front, there are some unique markers used in assessment. We look at various options to assess immune balance—specifically the balance between the TH1 and TH2 sides of the immune system. We can actually measure the cytokines produced by these two sides and measure a ratio between them.

There is also an array of specialized tests available, and I've narrowed them down to the more essential. As a general rule, there's no reason to look at laboratory tests if they're not going to change your course of action.

Some additional key tests I use include:

Antidiuretic Hormone (ADH): This is very common in people with chronic inflammation, especially when it is being underproduced. It's a hormone that tells the kidneys to properly hold onto water. When we're underproducing this important hormone, water "goes right through us." People will say they urinate a lot, drink a lot, urinate a lot, drink a lot, but never feel properly hydrated. This happens because, in essence, the brain is inflamed, allowing for hormone dysregulation.

Matrix Metalloproteinase 9 (MMP-9): This is associated with inflammation and a lack of proper integrity of the gut lining and respiratory tract. There's a pretty good correlation between elevated MMP-9 and gut and respiratory tract inflammation.

Melanocyte-Stimulating Hormone (MSH): This is very important in my opinion. MSH is a pituitary hormone that hasn't been given nearly enough credit. We don't learn much about it in medical school—I didn't forty years ago, and the med students I work with today aren't getting much more information. But it's a very important hormone that helps modulate the immune system, reduce inflammation, and promote healing. It also has antimicrobial properties for warding off infection. Very commonly, when we measure MSH, it's low, and we have very specific treatments for that.

Transforming Growth Factor Beta 1 (TGF-β1): This is an important measurement associated with inflammation that results from immune imbalance. When the TH1/TReg side is underactive and the TH2/TH17 side is overactive, TGF-β1 correlates with the runaway inflammation from that overactive side of the immune system. This gives us a good idea of the degree of inflammation resulting from immune imbalance. Keep in mind that a single test, such as an elevated TGF-B1, can be misleading by itself. We need to step back and take a big-picture view of all the lab results, the patient's symptoms, and more.

Understanding the immune system can be challenging. To try to simplify these pathways, we'll put it this way: TH1—fights viruses and intracellular bacteria, Treg—suppresses and regulates immune responses, TH2—defense against parasites + allergy responses, and TH17—defense against extracellular bacteria and fungi—more proinflammatory and autoimmune associated.

C-Reactive Protein (Cardiac): This measures inflammation in the lining of the arteries.

Ferritin: This measures the body's iron stores. Many of us, especially men, have iron levels that are much too high. In large part, we haven't been properly educated about the damaging effects of holding onto too much iron. Like an old I-beam at a steel mill scrapyard, iron rusts in our bodies too, causing oxidative stress. If we have more iron than we need, our body has to use its antioxidant capacity to neutralize that oxidative stress. This is commonly too high, especially in men or women who don't menstruate, and it's a health hazard. We can easily remedy this by donating blood to lower ferritin levels.

Fibrinogen Antigen: When elevated, this is associated with clotting risk due to chronic inflammation.

There are additional labs that I will commonly include, but they are considered individually depending on patient presentation and history. One example is the fasting leptin level in patients where leptin resistance is suspected. Chronic inflammation commonly causes leptin resistance, which can contribute to difficulty losing weight as well as difficulty fighting inflammation. As a side note, I frequently consider GLP-1 microdosing for those patients as part of a comprehensive protocol to treat chronic inflammation. As with most any medication, the poison is in the dose. Proper, judicious use of GLP-1 peptides can be extremely beneficial as a means to an end. The hope is that the patient will not have to stay on them long-term.

With all this laboratory information, I can accurately outline each patient's needs—from insulin resistance and metabolic disease to inflammation and the whole spectrum of what we address. I use these laboratory results to guide my recommended therapies and outline a treatment plan. Typically, after three to four months, I reassess and remeasure the abnormal labs. This allows us to accurately see what our interventions are doing and continue making modifications to the treatment regimen so we can continue to fine-tune and optimize health.

The key is that this is an ongoing process of assessment, treatment, and refinement based on objective laboratory data combined with clinical symptoms and patient response.

Inflammation-Friendly Lifestyle Changes

Looking back, we see a God-given health recommendation from the 1830s—seasonal eating by necessity. Things were, of course, different back then, but the principle still holds. If all people had during a particular winter was elk jerky, then that's what they consumed. Toward the top of the pyramid are grains—and I believe they're mentioned last (at the top) for good reason. Grains are fairly hard to digest, high in carbohydrates, and can help stimulate fat storage. Historically, people ate seasonal produce and even sweet fruits like apples in the fall, then grains during the winter to help put on fat to survive a little easier. Unfortunately, many of our modern grains are simply not what they used to be. They have been genetically modified, they're commonly harvested with glyphosate (Round-Up), and are not like the original ancient grains that our ancestors used. Making things worse, we typically don't process those grains the way our ancestors did, such as soaking and fermenting them, like with sourdough fermentation. Heirloom/ancient grains processed the way nature intended are less inflammatory and insulinogenic (insulin-stimulating).

The day and age we live in now is very different, but I still think the God-given food pyramid essentially outlines what we know as the Mediterranean diet—the most anti-inflammatory, heart-healthy type of diet available. It emphasizes lots of produce, vegetables, fruits, healthy fats like olive oil, and meats sparingly.

In my practice, I commonly start patients out, at least initially, on a low-lectin diet that avoids grains, sugars, processed foods, all beans, lentils, other legumes, some nuts and seeds, all dairy that contains the A1 protein, and specific vegetables such as tomatoes, squash, and bell peppers. Lectins are protein particles found in plants and their seeds, and they're there to protect the plant and its seeds so they can survive and have progeny. But they tend to be inflammatory, especially if a gut lining is already compromised and leaky.

A low-lectin diet can facilitate healing of the gut lining. Even nightshade vegetables, which many of us love—peppers, tomatoes, and potatoes—can be fairly high in lectins and inflammatory. So there might be a period of time when we need to consider a low-lectin diet, at least for the gut-healing phase.

But long-term, my intention is not to keep patients on such a restrictive diet. The goal is to eventually reintroduce some of those lectin-containing foods: nightshades, certain grains. For example, white sourdough is probably the least inflammatory bread we can consume (especially if it comes from an ancient/heirloom/organic source to begin with), assuming someone isn't very sensitive to gluten.

I'll also commonly test for gluten sensitivity because many of my patients with chronic inflammatory response syndrome have gluten issues and need to avoid gluten—in some cases long-term. Actually, I'm one of those who, fortunately, found out many years ago that I'm gluten sensitive, as are all of my siblings (an interesting genetic component).

The Long-Term Perspective

We should notice that Diet Coke or Twinkies aren't mentioned anywhere in that God-given food pyramid.

Diet Coke and Twinkies are not part of the God-given food pyramid.

When patients ask, often with some dismay, "Do I have to eat this way forever?" The answer is no. Once we correct things—once we treat the immune imbalance and chronic inflammation and optimize mitochondrial health—we're metabolically in a good place (metabolically flexible) and can tolerate those indiscretions. (Although Twinkies really aren't a great idea any time.)

In backcountry skiing, we use the term "earn your turns," as you need to hike up to ski down. Well, we can earn those diet indiscretions in a similar fashion, but it's a long process for many of us to get to the point where those dalliances won't be damaging. We can get there, however, and I think that gives my patients hope that we don't have to necessarily consider such a restrictive diet for the long haul. Lifestyle balance is the goal.

The Critical Role of Restorative Sleep and Exercise

We discuss it throughout this book—restorative sleep is incredibly critical and very commonly is not what it should be as we age. The pineal gland shrinks, and this gland is what controls our circadian rhythms. Fortunately, my favorite peptide can consistently restore its function. (More on this in the next chapter). It's a very anti-aging peptide that can often help restore those circadian rhythms by working through and "resetting" the pineal gland.

But sleep is ever so critical, and it's often not a matter of just wishing it would be better. A lot of my patients will try everything they can find online for sleep hygiene and sleep restoration, and those things help, but in many instances, poor sleep habits are often not easy to correct.

We recommend all those sleep hygiene techniques: the type of light we're exposed to in the evening, the temperature of our ambient environment in the evening, avoidance of stimulating blue light from screens. That all makes a big difference, but often it takes more intervention (dedicated commitment) than just basic measures to restore sleep.

Exercise is equally important in addressing chronic inflammation (or, even better, avoiding it in the first place). The impact of doing nothing is enormous, exponentially worse than doing something and gaining benefit, even if it's small. In some cases, we need to start low and go slow, but we've got to start moving. It's just so therapeutic. Even if all someone can do to begin with is a short walk outdoors, it's a start. Then we build on that.

Here's a great example: My father-in-law lives in St. George, Utah, and he is ninety-six years old. He stays active, always out moving. He rides his bike several times a week and still participates—I don't know if "playing" is the right term at this point—with the softball team he's been part of for years. He doesn't run the bases anymore, but he'll stand up and bat, stand at first base, and at least participate and support the younger-aged group.

That's the kind of mindset we need to cultivate—staying engaged, staying active, adapting as we need to, but never giving up on movement and participation in life. It's about finding what you *can* do, not what you can't.

In addition to everything lifestyle-oriented we've touched on in this chapter, there is yet another powerful tool we can employ. It's time to pull back the curtain and introduce peptides. They're tiny, powerful, and revolutionary.

CHAPTER 10

A Peptides Primer

Peptides are not foreign drugs;
they are whispers of the body's own design.

Functional Medicine axiom

Peptides are the body's chain gang. These naturally occurring molecules are short-chain amino acids—the building blocks of proteins—linked together to play a fundamental role in numerous biological functions. Unlike full proteins, which can consist of hundreds of amino acids, peptides typically contain between two and fifty amino acids, allowing them to be more easily absorbed and utilized by cells. There are over 7,000 known peptides in the human body, each with its own specific function. Many peptides act as signaling molecules, helping cells communicate with one another, and they regulate a variety of processes, including hormone production, immune responses, and cellular regeneration.

In the context of healing, peptides are crucial because they can stimulate the body's natural repair mechanisms. Specific peptides are known to promote tissue regeneration, reduce inflammation, and improve collagen synthesis—key processes in wound healing and recovery from injury. For example, peptides like BPC-157 (nicknamed the Wolverine peptide, which is fifteen amino acids in length) and TB-500 have gained attention in both clinical and wellness settings for their potential to accelerate recovery in muscles, tendons, and even the gut lining.

Consider the following patient case:

Sarah Martinez, a forty-two-year-old marathon runner, developed chronic tendinitis in her Achilles tendon that hadn't responded to six months of conventional treatment, including rest, physical therapy, and anti-inflammatory medications. The persistent inflammation prevented proper tissue repair, keeping her sidelined from running.

Her sports medicine physician introduced an oral form of BPC-157, a peptide derived from a protective protein found in gastric juice. This peptide addressed her condition by activating specific growth factor receptors in the damaged tendon tissue. Within the first few weeks of treatment, Sarah noticed a significant reduction in pain and stiffness.

The BPC-157 worked through multiple complementary mechanisms: It promoted angiogenesis (formation of new blood vessels) to improve nutrient delivery to the injured area, enhanced fibroblast migration to rebuild collagen fibers, and modulated inflammatory cytokines to reduce swelling without completely suppressing the immune response needed for healing.

After three months of peptide therapy combined with gradual physical rehabilitation, Sarah's tendon showed substantial improvement on ultrasound imaging—the disorganized, thickened tissue had been replaced with more organized collagen fibers. She was able to return to running at 80 percent of her previous capacity, with continued improvement expected.

Unlike NSAIDs, which can actually impair tendon healing when used long-term, the peptide worked *with* Sarah's natural healing processes, targeting the specific cellular pathways needed for tissue regeneration without the systemic side effects of traditional medications.

Peptides offer a more precise and often safer approach to healing than some traditional pharmaceuticals.

By targeting specific pathways, peptides offer a more precise and often safer approach to healing than some traditional pharmaceuticals, making them a promising frontier in regenerative medicine.

One common example of peptides is collagen peptides (broken-down pieces of collagen), which many people take as a supplement for skin, joint, or hair health. Collagen is a protein. Collagen peptides are shorter amino acid chains derived from collagen. These peptides aren't primarily signaling molecules—they're more like raw materials that the body can use to build collagen. They may have some signaling capacity, but their main function is structural.

Another common example is insulin, the first peptide ever discovered. It was originally derived from animals, and some peptides, like Cerebrolysin (and its oral version CerebroPep), are still animal-derived (in this case, from pig brain tissue) and are used for neurological regeneration. However, most peptides used today for therapeutic purposes are made synthetically for consistency and safety to mimic the molecules our bodies naturally make.

Today, the peptide market is booming in large part thanks to the popularity of the GLP-1 peptides being used for weight loss. However, many of the oral peptides sold online (especially on platforms like Amazon) are not true peptides. Third-party testing often reveals that they're just unlinked amino acids, which means they won't function the same way as true peptides in your body. Moreover, biological engineering made manufactured peptides require chemical "capping" (adding a capping molecule to block unreacted amino groups) at their ends for stability and efficacy. Without this, their quality and effectiveness are greatly reduced.

Despite these concerns, peptides are remarkable molecules. One standout example is BPC-157, known for its powerful healing and anti-inflammatory properties. Unlike ibuprofen, which only temporarily suppresses inflammation, BPC-157 actively promotes tissue repair while also reducing inflammation—making it profoundly regenerative. As we age, our natural peptide production declines, which contributes to slower healing and chronic inflammation. Fortunately, using therapeutic high-quality peptides can help restore those levels, optimize healing, and support overall vitality.

How Peptides Function in the Body

Peptides are the body's master communicators, tiny chains of amino acids that carry critical messages between cells and tissues. When a peptide locks onto a cell's receptor, it triggers a cascade of activity—releasing hormones, activating immune cells, or initiating repair processes—all from a molecule sometimes just a few amino acids long.

Let's look at how they work:

1. Production
   - Peptides are synthesized within cells from amino acids, the building blocks of proteins.
   - Some peptides are produced by the body (endogenous), while others come from external sources like food or supplements (exogenous).
2. Release and transportation
   - Once synthesized, peptides are released into the bloodstream or surrounding tissues.
   - They travel through the body to reach their target cells or tissues.
3. Targeting and binding
   - Peptides act like keys, and target cells have specific receptors (locks) on their surfaces.
   - When a peptide binds to its specific receptor, it triggers a cascade of events inside the cell.
4. Cellular response
   - The binding of the peptide to the receptor initiates various cellular processes, including:
   - Gene expression and protein synthesis: Peptides can influence the production of specific proteins by regulating gene expression.
     - Hormone secretion: Some peptides act as hormones, stimulating the release of other hormones.

- Immune modulation: Peptides can modulate (balance) the activity of immune cells to fight infections or inflammation and prevent or fight cancer.
- Metabolic regulation: Certain peptides control appetite, blood sugar levels, and fat metabolism.
- Growth and repair: Peptides can promote cell division, regeneration, and tissue healing.

5. Degradation and recycling
   - After initiating their effects, peptides are broken down into their individual amino acids by enzymes.
   - These amino acids can then be reused by the body to build new proteins or peptides.

With a primer of how peptides work in the body, let's now examine how to use them to invigorate the body's natural ability to heal.

The Peptide Revolution

The use of peptides to optimize the body's natural healing has created a "peptide revolution" in regenerative medicine through peptide therapy.

Peptide therapy consists primarily of synthetic (human-made) peptides that augment what the body is already producing. By doing so, we can optimize the critical signaling to facilitate cells to improve their various functions. It is a great way to improve overall health and well-being.

Peptide therapy augments what the body is already producing.

So how does it work? Peptide therapy delivers synthetic peptides to the body to activate specific cell functions that improve metabolism, muscle growth, and skin health. Each peptide has a unique function. For example, growth hormone-releasing hormones and growth hormone-releasing peptides increase growth hormone production and secretion. This helps with cellular efficiency, which improves body composition and metabolism, strength, performance and recovery, healing, sleep architecture, and longevity. Other peptides, like GHK-Cu (a copper peptide), help the skin produce more collagen and elastin and reduce inflammation. These compounds are typically injected or taken orally and interact with receptors in the body to trigger beneficial responses over time.

Every one of these peptides has a unique outcome. A peptide that helps build muscle is different from a peptide meant to improve the health and elasticity of your skin. If you are keen on using anti-aging peptides to rejuvenate tired skin, a properly trained physician can connect you with something to regenerate aging collagen. If you want to lose weight or gain muscle mass, there is a peptide that raises growth hormone levels, which result in those beneficial changes.

The science of peptides is simple yet powerful. Peptides serve as cellular signposts, guiding your body's processes in specific directions. They point cells toward growth, repair, or regulation, ensuring biological traffic flows where it is needed most.

Benefits of Peptide Therapy

The advantages of peptide therapy are manifold, contingent on the category of peptides used. Some of the most common benefits people report are:

Improved Skin Health: Peptides can be beneficial for the skin, as they help smooth wrinkles and fine lines by promoting collagen production. Collagen is a protein that helps your skin maintain firmness and a healthy appearance. Collagen naturally decreases as we age, causing lines and wrinkles to appear in the skin. This can be reversed by increasing collagen synthesis with the help of peptide therapy.

Muscle Building: People in sports or fitness fields use peptides to achieve a faster muscle-building process. Growth hormone, on the other hand, helps build bigger, stronger muscles.

Fat Burning: Peptides boost metabolism, which helps burn fat. Some specific peptides enhance metabolic rate, which increases calorie burning and fat oxidation. This process goes on to help our bodies efficiently use stored fat for energy.

Better Quality Sleep: Getting proper sleep, especially deep and REM sleep, drives repair, regeneration, and optimization of body and mind. Peptides, such as Epitalon and growth hormone secretagogue peptides, improve sleep quantity and quality.

Rapid Healing: Peptides, such as BPC 157, assist in healing and recovery from injury and everyday routines. It can make a great choice for athletes or those recovering from surgery.

Risks and Side Effects of Peptide Therapy

There are potential risks to any medical treatment, and peptide therapy is no different. As a rule, peptides are very safe compared to many pharmaceutical drugs. Before beginning peptide therapy, however, it is important to become familiar with potential side effects. These include:

Redness or Irritation: Some people may have slight redness and swelling at the site of injection.

Peptides Increase Appetite: Some peptides, especially some of those that promote growth hormones, may increase feelings of hunger. Water retention may also occur when using peptides that increase growth hormone levels. It's too soon to say what other symptoms might be directly related to peptide therapy, but fatigue or lightheadedness are possible.

Results from Peptide Therapy

Peptide therapy results vary from one individual to another. For some, it takes just a few weeks to experience positive results, while others may take a little longer before change becomes evident. It will also vary depending on the nature of peptides utilized and their general state of health.

Peptide therapy is most used in the modulation of:

Younger Looking Skin: A lot of people find that their skin appears firmer or healthier after beginning peptide treatment.

Build/Heal: Those who are using peptides to build muscle can expect more muscle and greater overall strength, while others significantly facilitate healing.

Weight Loss: Over a period of time: Certain peptides promote fat burning, also helping in losing excess weight.

Increased Energy Levels: Patients typically note better energy and are more refreshed when starting peptide therapy.

Optimal Sleep Restoration: As previously mentioned, some peptides greatly enhance restorative sleep.

Immunomodulation: Peptides such as Thymogen Alpha 1, TB4 Frag, and KPV are quite immunomodulating (balancing).

The key takeaway is that peptide therapy functions optimally when integrated into a comprehensive healthy lifestyle, with daily activity and optimized sleep.

Peptide Therapy: Before and After

Peptide therapy before and after comparisons show improved energy with associated improved fat burning and maintenance of lean muscle mass, improved sleep, improvement in mental clarity and focus, improved mood, and more resilience to stress. People looking for peptide weight loss often report slimmer waistlines, better energy, and reduced cravings. Visual changes can include a healthier complexion, tighter skin, and more toned body contours. In a clinical setting, I frequently use peptides as part of a comprehensive protocol to treat chronic inflammation, and in those cases, the before and after outcomes can be quite dramatic. Of course, results depend on the peptides used and lifestyle habits like sleep, nutrition, exercise, and meditative/spiritual practices.

Five Powerful Peptides

In my practice, I commonly use a host of five powerful peptides, with a very positive impact on my patients. Here are those key players' clinical applications and their benefits.

1 BPC-157 (Body Protective Compound 1-57)

What it is

A synthetic peptide found naturally in and derived from the stomach's gastric juices.

Structure

Fifteen amino acids in length

Primary Functions

- Tissue healing and regeneration throughout the body
- Simultaneous inflammation reduction
- Stimulates cell proliferation and angiogenesis (new blood vessel formation)

Key Benefits

Musculoskeletal: Accelerates healing of muscles, tendons, ligaments, bones, and joints

Gastrointestinal: Profoundly anti-inflammatory in the GI tract, promotes gut lining healing, and improves overall gut health

Neurological: Neuroprotective properties that shield nerve cells from damage caused by stroke or spinal cord injury

Athletic Performance: Enhances muscle growth and strength, making it popular in bodybuilding and athletics

Wound Healing: Accelerates general wound healing processes

(2) Epithalon (Epitalon)

What it is

A synthetic peptide that mimics a natural pineal gland hormone. Epitalon is widely believed to regulate telomerase production, an enzyme linked to cellular aging and longevity.

Structure

Bioregulatory peptide

Primary Functions

- Anti-aging through telomere lengthening
- Sleep and immune system enhancement
- Mortality reduction

Key Benefits

Longevity: Lengthens telomeres (DNA protective caps that influence aging rate), slowing the aging process and decreasing mortality

Clinical Evidence: A Russian study of 80-plus-year-old retired coal miners showed 80 percent mortality in the control group vs. 20 percent in the Epithalon group over six years (treatment: two weeks every six months)

Antioxidant Support: Normalizes antioxidant pathways, increases glutathione peroxidase activity, reduces lipid oxidation

Sleep Quality: Improves pineal gland function, normalizes circadian rhythms and melatonin production, enhances deep sleep and REM sleep

Immune Function: Strengthens both cellular and humoral immunity through improved thymus gland function

Metabolic Health: Improves insulin sensitivity, helps with metabolic syndrome and prediabetes

Cardiovascular: Decreases LDL cholesterol, raises HDL cholesterol, improves overall lipid profiles

Additional Benefits: Tissue repair, anti-tumor/anti-cancer activity, improved sex hormone regulation

3 TB-4 Fragment

What it is

A shortened version of a naturally occurring peptide that promotes tissue repair, reduces inflammation, and supports wound healing throughout the body.

Structure

Fragment of TB-500 (TB-4) peptide, a shorter amino acid chain

Primary Functions

- Tissue regeneration and immune system modulation
- Oral bioavailability (unlike TB-500)

Key Benefits

Immune Balance: Balances immune system by improving TH1/T-regulatory cell function, addressing chronic inflammation

Bioavailability: Superior oral absorption compared to injectable TB-500

Neurological: Supports cognitive function

Gastrointestinal: Protects the GI barrier

Mental Health: Promotes mood stability

Cardiovascular: Provides heart protection

General Wellness: Promotes overall well-being

4 Thymogen Alpha-1

What it is

A thymus-derived peptide that supports immune system function by helping regulate T-cell activity and maintaining proper immune response balance.

Structure

Synergistic blend of two separate bioregulatory dipeptides (two amino acids each)

Primary Functions

- Immune system modulation and enhancement
- Thymus gland restoration

Key Benefits

Immune Enhancement: Increases white blood cell activity and normalizes lymphocyte counts

Antimicrobial: Potent antimicrobial activity

Thymus Function: Boosts and restores thymus gland function (unique as a thymus-derived peptide)

Anti-Aging: Reduces age-related cellular degeneration

Inflammation: Acts as a "chaperoning peptide" to correct and reduce inflammation

Cancer Prevention: Lowers cancer risk

(5) KPV

What it is

A tripeptide with potent anti-inflammatory properties that helps modulate immune responses and protect the gut lining from inflammatory damage.

Structure

Tripeptide (three amino acids)—terminal fragment of alpha melanocyte-stimulating hormone

Primary Functions

- Potent anti-inflammatory action
- Multiple administration routes (oral, subcutaneous, topical)

Key Benefits

Safety Profile: No notable side effects

Versatile Delivery: Works through multiple administration methods

Anti-Inflammatory: Treats various inflammatory conditions, including IBD, asthma, eczema, and psoriasis

Antimicrobial: Provides antimicrobial effects

Skin Health: Improves overall skin health and wound healing

UV Protection: Enhances tanning ability and reduces burn risk, providing natural UV protection

Clinical Applications: Well-studied for topical psoriasis treatment

Clinical Considerations

All told, these peptides bring a diverse range of therapeutic applications, from tissue regeneration and anti-aging to immune modulation and inflammation control. Each offers unique mechanisms of action and can be used individually or in combination based on specific therapeutic goals. In addition, the oral bioavailability of several of these peptides makes them particularly attractive because of their ease of use and safety profile.

What does patient response look like? As with most medical applications, some patients respond differently to peptides, but overall, we see dramatic improvement in whole-body health. Some peptides have effects that people notice almost immediately, while others work more subtly in the background over time. One that tends to produce quicker results is **Epitalon**, which works through the pineal gland to help normalize its function. It can be taken orally, and I typically recommend dosing one capsule twice a day. It's not like a pharmaceutical that makes you drowsy during the day (rarely reported), but many patients report improved sleep quality and overall well-being within days of starting this peptide.

Other peptides, like **BPC-157**, are more gradual in their effects. **BPC-157** is a healing peptide that helps reduce inflammation and support tissue repair. Most people who take it won't feel anything right away, but over time—especially after a month or two—they often realize that nagging issues, like shoulder pain, have significantly improved. I see this commonly in men over age forty-five, many of whom have dealt with chronic shoulder issues at some point.

KPV is another peptide that works behind the scenes. People who begin taking it may not notice immediate effects, but it can help reduce systemic inflammation and improve conditions like asthma, allergies, eczema, psoriasis, and even sensitivity to sunburn. It also plays a unique role in immune regulation. I often prescribe it to patients with low levels of **melanocyte-stimulating hormone (MSH)**. In about 80 percent of these cases, a nasal culture reveals a specific form of staph bacteria—**MARCoNS**—which produces toxins that suppress pituitary MSH production.

This creates a cycle where low MSH allows the bacteria to thrive, which in turn keeps MSH levels suppressed. By supplementing with KPV, we can help break that cycle. Over three to six months, we usually see MSH levels rise again. Once those levels are sufficient, the body can maintain control over the bacteria without needing continued peptide support.

Other peptides like **TB-500 (or TB4-FRAG**) and **Thymogen Alpha-1** also work in this immunomodulating (adjusting to the appropriate level, like a thermostat) and regenerative space. Thymogen Alpha-1 may not produce noticeable effects right away, but it helps balance the body's immune response. TB4-FRAg, much like BPC-157, supports healing and tissue repair, making these two peptides a great combination for chronic injuries or recovery.

For maximum therapeutic benefit, we can also combine multiple peptides. When treating chronic inflammatory response syndrome, I typically recommend several peptides simultaneously, though the specific combination depends on individual lab results.

One important marker we monitor is transforming growth factor beta-1 (TGF-β1). If this marker of inflammation is elevated, it suggests immune imbalance. When TGF-β1 is elevated above normal ranges, I'll include the peptides Thymogen Alpha 1 and TB4 Frag in the protocol along with LDN (low-dose naltrexone) for their immunomodulating effect. (See *Transforming Growth Factor Beta 1 (TGF-β1)* in the previous chapter.)

The dosing strategy depends on severity: If TGF-β1 exceeds 10,000, I increase the immunomodulating peptides to twice daily instead of once daily. There is definitely an art to determining the right combination, dosages, and timing intervals. Ultimately, treatment duration varies significantly by individual and peptide type. In most cases, as soon as certain inflammatory markers and hormone levels have normalized, the respective peptides can be discontinued. For example:

Epitalon often resets pineal gland function for a prolonged period of time. Some studies suggest just two weeks every six months for anti-aging benefits. Many patients maintain improved sleep even after discontinuing this peptide. With that in mind, I suggest taking a four-week course or so whenever someone feels like they need a sleep reset. For those who love tracking sleep data, that information can help dictate when another reset course of Epitalon is warranted.

These peptides serve as tools to restore normal function rather than forming lifelong dependencies as compared to pharmaceutical prescriptions. I keep patients on protocols long enough to achieve and confirm the targeted corrections, then we reassess and adjust accordingly to maintain progress toward optimal health. In practice, this can look like:

- Immunomodulating peptides can be discontinued once follow-up blood work confirms an immune system has returned to healthy levels.
- KPV is discontinued once the body's own melanocyte-stimulating hormone production normalizes.

A Look Inside Peptides

One particular question about peptides that I hear from nearly every patient, in one form or another, is, "What's going on in there?"

Peptides in our bodies are doing their thing. At some point, do they "lose their power?" Do we need to step in with some help?

We don't have complete answers to why the natural peptides our bodies produce wane with age, but several factors contribute to this decline. For one, age-related decline affects peptides produced by the pineal and thymus glands. These glands naturally become less healthy over time, producing fewer peptides like epithalamin, thymosin alpha-1, and thymulin. Using supplemental peptides like Epitalon can help restore functionality to these glands.

Chronic inflammation creates a different problem. Brain inflammation disrupts the pituitary gland's production of melanocyte-stimulating hormone, which isn't necessarily age-related but inflammation-driven. When the pituitary doesn't produce enough of this hormone, certain staph bacteria can overgrow in the nose and sinuses. This creates a vicious cycle where the bacteria further suppress hormone production, trapping us in a self-perpetuating problem that requires intervention.

The complexity deepens when you consider that epithalamin has been shown to open DNA strands, making them more receptive to other peptides. Once dysregulation begins, systems start cascading downward. I envision this as a domino effect, starting with genetic predisposition toward immune imbalance. The immune system's regulatory side becomes underactive while the inflammatory side becomes overactive. This opens the door for inflammation and sets dominoes falling in different patterns for each person.

The brain becomes inflamed, creating more dysregulation. The gut, closely connected to immune function, gets insulted early in this process. Leaky gut becomes leakier, inflammation increases, and dysregulation worsens. Eventually, mitochondria suffer from all the downstream inflammation. When cellular batteries aren't recharging properly, no cells function optimally, and the situation deteriorates further into a cycle of chronic inflammation that includes the cell danger response. The mitochondrial dysfunction at the end of this cascade feeds back to the beginning, perpetuating the cycle. This is why I feel simultaneous intervention works best: immunomodulation, inflammation treatment, gut healing, and mitochondrial optimization. These specific blood markers guide our interventions and address all these areas together for the best chance of restoring optimal health.

AN INTERESTING SIDE NOTE

With so many benefits for optimized health, peptides are, for the moment, still flying under the radar. Traditional medicine tends to resist early adoption of new treatments. Functional medicine practitioners are much more likely to be early adopters, keeping their ears to the ground for cutting-edge, transformative therapies. They're typically the ones discovering and integrating these approaches into their practices first.

Traditional medical practices currently don't discuss peptides much, even though they're already using them without realizing it. GLP-1 medications, which are extremely popular and used in practices nationwide and globally, are actually peptides. Many practitioners don't recognize this, and even if they do, they lack knowledge about other peptides and their therapeutic potential. But the standard of care often means following established protocols without questioning the status quo. This approach stifles innovation, change, and improvement in medical treatment.

How Peptides Heal Inflammation

Let's look more closely at how peptides signal the body to heal and reduce inflammation and how they work at the cellular level to reduce inflammation by modulating the immune system's response.

By targeting the underlying causes of chronic inflammation, peptides can help reduce pain, repair tissue damage, and improve overall immune function. Peptides function as cellular communication molecules, acting as signaling messengers that trigger cascades of intracellular responses through a process called signal transduction. The process begins with binding. Peptides, also called ligands, bind to specific receptors on target cell surfaces. These receptors interact with specific chemical messages, ensuring signal specificity.

There are three major categories of cell surface peptide receptors: G protein-coupled receptors, enzyme-coupled receptors, and ion channel-coupled receptors. Once the peptide binds, receptor activation occurs. The receptor changes shape and activates associated signaling pathways. I think of this as a lock-and-key mechanism—the key finds the lock, and once it enters, it triggers a response and opens the door. Consider the following graphic:

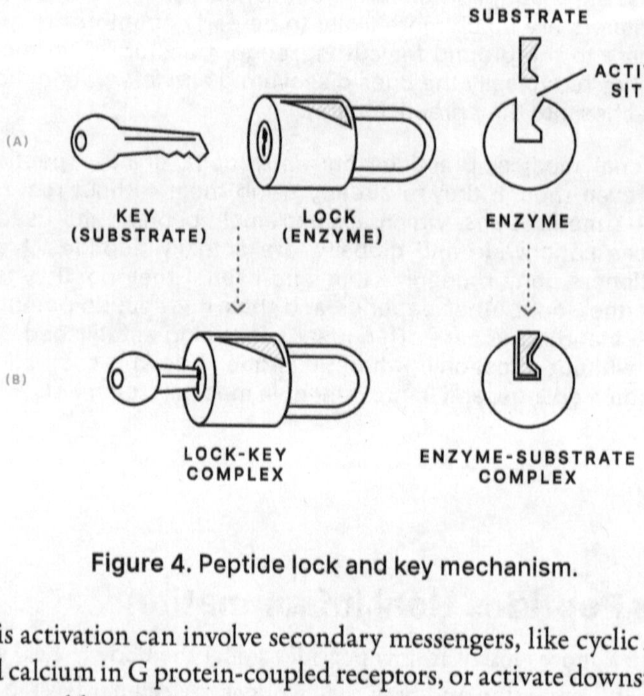

Figure 4. Peptide lock and key mechanism.

This activation can involve secondary messengers, like cyclic AMP and calcium in G protein-coupled receptors, or activate downstream effectors like PI3K in enzyme-coupled receptors. The details get complex, but the key point is that it triggers a cascade of changes and signals. The activation of these pathways leads to specific cellular responses such as growth, differentiation, and metabolism, which involve energy production through mitochondrial function and highly specific peptide-receptor interactions.

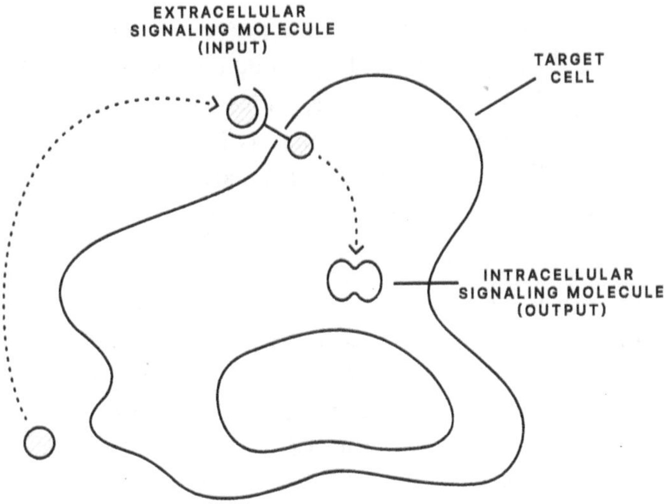

Figure 5. Peptide signaling (No. 1).

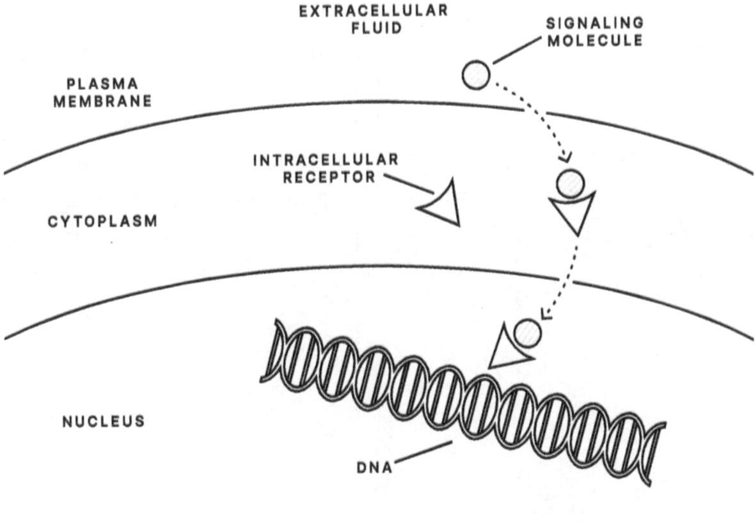

Figure 6. Peptide signaling (No. 2).

Examples of peptide signaling include peptide hormones that regulate metabolism, growth, and reproduction. Neurotransmitters transmit signals between neurons, influencing mood, learning, and memory. Growth factors promote cell growth, proliferation, and healing—BPC-157 definitely stimulates growth factors in this capacity.

> **"For years I lived in cycles of pain and slow recovery, never truly bouncing back. When I began BPC-157 and TB4 Frag, it felt like my body remembered how to heal. The pain eased, my energy returned, and for the first time in years, I could imagine a future of health instead of limitation."**
>
> PATIENT TESTIMONIAL

While the process is far from simple, it starts with that crucial first step: The peptide binds to its receptor, and depending on the situation, this triggers a cascade of other cellular events.

With some understanding of how peptides function at the cellular level—from their natural production and age-related decline to their specific receptor interactions and signaling cascades—we can explore the practical application of this knowledge. Next, we'll examine how to strategically use peptides alongside targeted supplements and dietary interventions to optimize health outcomes and address specific therapeutic goals.

CHAPTER 11

A Peptides Approach to Optimizing Health

From repairing injuries and reducing inflammation to supporting weight loss and potentially slowing aging, peptides are redefining how we approach health.

Dr. Mark Hyman

Peptides aren't magic... but they're close. When patients ask me, "What's going on in there?" about peptides, a common follow-up question is: "If peptides are already in our bodies, doing their thing, isn't that good enough?" The answer is that while they are already in our bodies, they are not at the levels that they once were when we were young and vibrant. The truth is, we can all benefit from restoring those more youthful levels of these miraculous molecules as part of a longevity-focused health optimization regimen.

Whether we're treating chronic inflammatory response syndrome, managing chronic inflammation, or simply pursuing optimal health, the foundation (digestive, immune, nervous, and mitochondrial) remains remarkably consistent. The game-changer in my practice has been the integration of peptides into treatment regimens. Before incorporating these miraculous molecules, achieving the results patients hoped for was significantly more challenging. Peptides provide that crucial bridge, taking us from good to better to our next level-best!

The latest dietary advice, life-changing exercise routines, and powerful vitamins are available everywhere—from online videos to pharmacy counters. But all of that only goes so far unless you fully commit. For example, the Mediterranean diet is excellent, but unless you consistently source the right ingredients, diligently prepare meals, and maintain strict adherence, you're leaving the benefits on the table. Achieving the level of compliance needed for optimal results requires commitment, effort, and consistency.

So how do we build a comprehensive health regimen? There are three steps:

1. First and foremost, we need desire. Without it, change simply won't happen.
2. Next, there also must be a plan, ideally written or otherwise recorded.
3. And the final step is to compile a list of goals, along with the accountability steps to reach them.

The **positive mindset** component—visualizing the health changes you hope to achieve—provides the final piece of this comprehensive approach.

A comprehensive health regimen takes you from the anti-inflammatory start line to the mitochondrial function finish line.

With that in place, it's off to the optimized health races, from an anti-inflammatory diet start line to the gut-healing homestretch and the mitochondrial function finish line.

Integrative Protocols for Optimal Health

This is where peptides change everything. When you add a peptide element to your foundational diet and exercise protocol, you get that additional boost needed to reach optimal health. I emphasize dietary improvements to all my patients, but I recognize that perfect adherence is unrealistic (which is not an excuse to not give it our best effort). Nobody executes a diet flawlessly. To that end, I give patients flexibility while encouraging them to aim high, keep making improvements, and persist through setbacks. The addition of peptides to those foundational treatments makes a transformative difference.

What makes this approach so effective isn't any single intervention, but rather the synergistic effect of addressing multiple systems simultaneously. When you combine optimized nutrition, strategic fasting, restorative sleep, targeted supplementation, and cutting-edge peptide therapy, you create conditions where the body can heal itself and achieve levels of health that seemed impossible with conventional approaches alone.

Optimized Nutrition

In the thick of my competitive athletic years, I discovered that strict ketogenic protocols could deliver remarkable mitochondrial enhancement for endurance performance. For years, I maintained very rigid adherence and saw excellent results. Once metabolic flexibility and enhanced mitochondrial function have been optimized, I have found that it's not as critical to maintain prolonged ketosis, which allows for more dietary flexibility. I still recommend that many of my patients consider a healthy version of a ketogenic diet, especially for those who suffer from significant mitochondrial dysfunction (those with slow metabolism).

Today, I commonly recommend an anti-inflammatory approach centered around the Mediterranean diet. For patients showing evidence or symptoms of leaky gut, I suggest a low-lectin diet initially—avoiding grains, sugars, processed foods, all legumes, nightshade vegetables, and some nuts and seeds. However, this restriction isn't necessary for everyone. Even for those who do need it, once the gut lining improves through following a low-lectin, Mediterranean, low-carb approach, they can gradually reintroduce restricted foods.

My current recommendations exist on a spectrum. On the more relaxed end, I might suggest a modified paleo approach that eliminates grains and sugars while allowing A2 dairy products (dairy containing beta-casein protein from specifically bred cows, goats, and sheep). This differentiates my recommendations from more restrictive autoimmune diets that eliminate all dairy—a restriction I consider unnecessarily limiting. (A2-derived dairy products are perfectly acceptable in my view.)

Strategic Fasting

I recommend strategic or intermittent fasting—an eating pattern based on time limits each day—for virtually everyone, especially when enhancing mitochondrial health. Solid evidence supports incorporating intermittent fasting.[39] That said, fasting isn't easy, especially for the uninitiated.

I recommend trying to fast five out of seven days weekly, allowing flexibility for social dining occasions when appropriate. The easiest intermittent fasting method for most people is to have breakfast later in the day or skip it entirely. (I use this modified adage constantly in my practice: "Breakfast is the most important meal of the day" is simply missing the words "to skip.") This typically means a 16-hour fast from dinner until your next meal.

In addition, I advise patients to stop eating two to three hours before going to sleep. For example, if bedtime is 11 p.m., plan to finish eating by 8 p.m. That starts the clock for a 16-hour fast ending at noon the next day. Of course, some people might prefer to finish eating early in the afternoon, starting their clock differently and skipping dinner, but this can be socially difficult for most people. Family dinner time has significant social benefits and helps maintain close family connections.

Here's how I employed fasting in competition. Over a seven-year stretch of strict ketogenic adherence, I consistently exercised in a fasted state to force mitochondrial adaptation. This doesn't feel good initially—you feel weaker—but it creates fuel flexibility and improves fat-burning capacity. On large training days and during races, I would use carbohydrates, but they felt like superfuel because I had forced mitochondrial adaptation through a ketogenic diet, intermittent fasting, and fasted exercise. I initially implemented these strategies during the off-season (October to February) because the initial negative performance impact was noticeable. Your high-end performance suffers, but you're building a low-end endurance base. That approach absolutely works.

I still recommend hydration and electrolytes during exercise but purposely avoiding fueling beforehand because of the mitochondrial benefit. Remember: There's no wrong way to approach intermittent fasting. When people struggle with fasting, it reveals that their mitochondria aren't fat-adapted or fuel-flexible—a common condition in our society that indicates optimization is needed.

Restorative Sleep

Whether enhancing mitochondria or treating chronic inflammation, restorative sleep is a non-negotiable. Restorative sleep encompasses sleep hygiene, optimizing the ambient environment with dimmed lights, avoiding blue light, controlling the temperature, and purposely viewing morning sunlight to reset circadian rhythms.

The Epitalon peptide discussed earlier represents a breakthrough in this area. Approximately 90 percent of my patients have reported improved sleep depth after their first day or two of supplementation. In fact, many patients who track sleep with smartwatches or Oura rings can see the improvement immediately in their sleep and post-exercise/recovery data—the difference is remarkable.

Targeted Supplementation

Essential Fatty Acids

You cannot achieve optimal health or win the battle against inflammation while being omega-deficient. Essential fats, including omega fish oils, typically represent my number one supplement recommendation. They are called "essential" for a reason! More than 68 percent of American adults and 95 percent of children are omega-3 deficient.[40] Consider testing your omega index with an OmegaQuant test. It's a home "finger prick" test and is fairly inexpensive. When we test, supplement, and then retest, we are much more likely to comply and thereby glean the most benefit from supplementation.

The active ingredients in omega-3 fatty acids—EPA and DHA—should total 1,500 to 2,000 milligrams for daily dosing maintenance. And since fats integrate into cells over months, if you miss a daily dose, make it up. For example, if your maintenance dose is two capsules daily, ensure you take fourteen capsules weekly.

For those new to omega supplementation, I recommend loading (a short phase of taking a higher than normal dose) by doubling the dose for six to eight weeks before dropping to maintenance levels. For those regularly eating cold water fatty fish, like wild-caught salmon, kipper snacks, or sardines—good on ya! You may not need supplementation. Keep up the good work.

To remember optimal fish choices, I use the SMASH acronym: salmon, mackerel, anchovies, sardines, and herring.

It is also worth mentioning phospholipids and choline. Phospholipids are critical fats that are commonly overlooked in cellular membrane optimization. Among the most notable is phosphatidylcholine, which supports acetylcholine—the neurotransmitter of the parasympathetic nervous system's restorative, rest, and digest side (the yang to the yin).

Organic sunflower lecithin powder provides an inexpensive phospholipid source—about a tablespoon several times weekly delivers adequate phospholipids at much lower cost than pure phosphatidylcholine. The only drawback is it doesn't mix well in cold beverages. Hot tip: Combine sunflower lecithin with naturally sweetened chocolate whey protein and unsweetened almond milk and mix in a blender or shaker bottle.

With choline (which many people don't get enough of and genetically require more), egg yolks represent the richest source, and those who regularly eat plenty of egg yolks may not need phospholipid supplementation.

Neuro-regeneration Supplements

Neuro-regeneration supplements are nutrients or compounds that are believed to **support the repair, regrowth, or protection of nerve cells** and their connections. The brain, being central to the nervous system, is invariably inflamed in chronic inflammatory conditions. Critical blood tests I administer to patients often reveal inadequate pituitary production of antidiuretic hormone and melanocyte-stimulating hormone (to name just two) due to brain inflammation. In other words, the pituitary gland may not make enough of certain important hormones, like those that help control water balance and skin pigment.

Curcumin

Curcumin, the active ingredient in turmeric, supports inflammation reduction and neuro-regeneration. Liposomal curcumin offers superior bioavailability and blood-brain barrier penetration compared to standard (non-liposomal) forms of curcumin. While perhaps not as critical for younger individuals, those over age forty who are concerned about brain health may benefit significantly from its broad anti-inflammatory and neuro-regenerative effects.

Methylene Blue

Methylene blue (introduced in Chapter Six) represents another fascinating molecule for mitochondrial enhancement and neuro-regeneration. Since the brain accounts for only 2 percent of our body weight but 20 percent of the body's ATP production, mitochondrial enhancers like methylene blue produce noticeable cognitive improvements in the brain's processing speed and focus. Many of my patients conditioned to stimulant medications like Adderall are able to successfully detach from them when starting methylene blue. Keep in mind, it is just more noticeable cognitively as it helps mitochondrial function throughout the body.

Immunomodulation Approach

Chronic inflammatory response syndrome's furthest upstream problem is a propensity for immune system imbalance. Blood tests, including transforming growth factor beta-one levels, guide our immunomodulation approach.

Low-dose naltrexone (LDN) serves as a cornerstone therapy treatment. Interestingly, naltrexone is an FDA-approved treatment for opioid addiction. We've discovered that even at very low doses, naltrexone causes the body to reflexively produce more endorphins. These endorphins provide immunomodulation while supporting mood and pain management—essentially the runner's high hormone produced artificially.

Immunomodulating peptides like **Thymogen** Alpha-1 and TB-4 Fragment complement this approach. Thymogen Alpha-1 calms overactive immune responses while improving underactive components. TB-4 Fragment enhances underactive immunity and promotes healing. LDN offers an affordable long-term preventive strategy for those with immune imbalance tendencies. I commonly recommend staying on LDN long-term for those with chronic inflammation propensity, even after I see that inflammation is squelched and the immune system is balanced. It can help keep us in proper immune balance and reduce the risk of the immune system going "wacky" again.

The **KPV peptide** offers targeted treatment for patients with chronic inflammation and low melanocyte-stimulating hormone levels—which is extremely common. KPV represents a terminal fragment of melanocyte-stimulating hormone itself. Low melanocyte-stimulating hormone levels typically correlates with antibiotic-resistant staph (MARCoNS) overgrowth. This creates a vicious cycle: staph produces toxins near the brain and pituitary, suppressing melanocyte-stimulating hormone production needed to fight the staph overgrowth.

KPV breaks this cycle by eliminating MARCoNS overgrowth. In my experience, four to six months of KPV treatment corrects this problem in approximately 80 percent of cases, restoring natural melanocyte hormone production and eliminating the need for continued KPV supplementation.

Gut-Healing Approach

Elevated TMAO (trimethylamine N-oxide) levels scream that gut lining permeability is severe. In these cases, I use aggressive gut-healing approaches, including Nitazoxanide combined with the peptide larazotide.

Nitazoxanide is a compound in the ivermectin family with antiparasitic, antiviral, immunomodulating properties and other benefits, including cancer treatment support.

Larazotide, on the other hand, blocks zonulin, a substance that breaks down the connections between digestive tract lining cells. By blocking this "glue breaker," we facilitate much more rapid healing. Matrix metalloproteinase-9 (MMP-9) elevation also suggests leaky gut and/or respiratory tract inflammation, though I typically reserve larazotide for elevated TMAO and MMP9 to facilitate gut healing, though this peptide heals throughout the body, not just the gut. Produced naturally in the stomach, BPC-157 demonstrates pronounced gut healing properties, especially when taken orally.

I also include diverse peptide fiber blends for those not consuming seven to nine daily vegetable servings (which is all of us). These blends support microbiome diversity and encourage the growth of microbes producing natural GLP-1 (our body's Ozempic) in the gut, supporting appetite control, weight management, gut lining healing, and reduction of inflammation.

Spore-based probiotics provide additional support, though fermented vegetables like sauerkraut, kimchi, and real pickles deliver higher spore-based probiotic doses plus postbiotics—the organic acids giving sauerkraut its tangy flavor—that protect and heal the gut lining. While approximately 50 percent of my patients wrinkle their noses at eating fermented vegetables, supplemental postbiotics like butyrate can provide short-term support until consistent prebiotic supplementation establishes natural postbiotic production.

Mitochondrial Enhancement Protocol

Beyond the foundational low-carb diet, intermittent fasting, restorative sleep, and fish oil, mitochondrial optimization (improving the health and function of our cells' "power plants") includes comprehensive multivitamins with ingredients like alpha lipoic acid, chromium, and acetyl-L-carnitine. CoQ10, or its active metabolite ubiquinol (for those over fifty), provides additional mitochondrial support.

Why is this important? Healthy mitochondria are essential for:

1. **Energy and stamina:** Tired or damaged mitochondria mean fatigue and poor endurance.
2. **Brain and nerve health:** The brain has a huge energy demand; poor mitochondrial function is linked to "brain fog," mood changes, and neurodegenerative diseases.
3. **Metabolic balance:** They regulate how your body burns fat, sugar, and oxygen.
4. **Aging and longevity:** Mitochondrial decline is a key factor in aging and age-related diseases.
5. **Immune and stress response:** Healthy mitochondria help cells respond to inflammation and oxidative stress.

NAD+ optimization represents another crucial component. This molecule becomes depleted with age and chronic inflammation, but we now have effective strategies to optimize the NAD+ to NADH ratio through precursor supplementation, liposomal NAD+ orally, and supportive compounds. Interestingly, bioflavonoids like quercetin and apigenin benefit mitochondria through NAD+ optimization. PQQ, urolithin A, and resveratrol—known for anti-aging benefits—provide their effects through NAD+ level optimization. In short, supporting NAD+ and mitochondrial health helps your cells make energy more efficiently, which can boost overall vitality, brain function, and healthy aging—all good things! Our overall health is directly proportional to our mitochondrial health.

In our medical spa, we offer NAD+ IV therapy as the most proven, aggressive mitochondrial reset strategy. This treatment proved invaluable during my own health challenges earlier this year when antibiotic-induced mitochondrial damage required aggressive intervention.

Exercise, particularly high-intensity interval training combined with resistance, hyperbaric oxygen, and aerobic work, ideally performed in a fasted state, completes the mitochondrial enhancement protocol.

This approach represents medicine's future—precision and personalized interventions that work with your body's natural healing mechanisms rather than simply suppressing symptoms. The result isn't just the absence of disease, but genuine vitality and optimal health that allows you to thrive at any age.

In essence, what I call Dr. Porter's Insulin Resistance Cure protocol is also my mitochondrial enhancement protocol, shared in this section, with an additional discussion on NAD+ enhancement strategies.

Comprehensive Metabolic Health and Recovery Protocol

This protocol addresses insulin resistance, metabolic syndrome, and chronic inflammatory conditions. Consult with healthcare providers before starting, especially for prescription medications and IV therapies, and monitor progress through appropriate lab work and clinical assessments. Expect to adjust dosages and timing based on response and tolerance levels.

Understanding the Conditions

Many health problems—ranging from blood sugar imbalances to chronic inflammation—share a common thread: When the body's energy systems and immune responses aren't working properly, multiple organs and systems can be affected. For example:

Insulin Resistance occurs when cells in muscles, fat, and the liver don't respond well to insulin and can't easily take up glucose from blood. The pancreas compensates by making more insulin, eventually leading to elevated blood sugar levels. This process has a strong association with mitochondrial dysfunction.

Insulin Resistance Syndrome (also called Metabolic Syndrome) includes high blood pressure, high cholesterol, type 2 diabetes, and obesity.

Chronic Inflammatory Response Syndrome includes persistent immune dysregulation, uncontrolled inflammation, and downstream dysfunction in multiple organ systems.

Core Protocol Elements (for insulin resistance/mitochondrial enhancement)

1. **Nutrition Foundation**
    - Anti-inflammatory diet: Mediterranean diet or modified paleo allowing dairy from goat, sheep, and Southern European cow sources (A2 casein-derived)
    - Low-carb Mediterranean approach (consider a ketogenic diet in those with insulin resistance/mitochondrial dysfunction)
    - Intermittent fasting
2. **Sleep Optimization**
    - Seven to eight hours of restorative sleep nightly
    - Consider Epitalon for sleep enhancement if needed
3. **Exercise Program (five to seven days per week)**—preferably in a fasted state
    - HIIT (High-Intensity Interval Training)
    - Resistance training
    - Aerobic exercise

4. **Essential Supplements**

   Supplement quality matters—choose pharmaceutical-grade products when possible.

   - Quality fish oil (if it causes fishy burps, it's rancid): EPA + DHA totaling 1,500–2,000mg/day for maintenance, but consider loading with double that amount for eight weeks if starting from scratch. These omega-3 fatty acids are called essential fatty acids for very good reason—they are *essential*!
   - Multivitamin: such as Mitocore (from OrthoMolecular) or similar for mitochondrial support (two to four daily)—a broad-spectrum multivitamin that includes methylated B-vitamins, chromium, alpha lipoic acid, acetyl L-carnitine, and other mitochondrial supporting ingredients
   - CoQ10: 200mg daily, or Ubiquinol 100mg daily if over age fifty. Berberine: 500mg twice daily with food (for blood sugar support for those with insulin resistance). Consider skipping on resistance exercise days.

   Brain and Neurological Support

   - Curcumin (liposomal form preferred)
   - Methylene Blue: 4–16 mg in the morning (mitochondrial enhancement)
   - Phospholipids: two quality eggs (with yolks) daily (on average) or sunflower lecithin powder
   - PQQ or Quercetin and Apigenin

   Inflammation Management

   - Pro-resolving mediators for inflammation and pain (typically recommended if pain persists despite other treatments)
   - KPV: For low MSH (melanocyte-stimulating hormone) levels, you may consider adding nano silver nasal spray as well

5. **Advanced NAD+ Optimization Strategies** (for those with significant mitochondrial dysfunction)

   Goal: Increase NAD+/NADH ratio

   Phase 1 (Month 1)

   - 5-Amino-1MQ: 50mg twice daily (currently research-only availability)

   Phase 2 (After Month 1, Choose One)

   - NAD+ IV Therapy: 750mg sessions, five treatments over two weeks (approximately three-hour sessions each)
   - NAD+ Subcutaneous Injections: 100mg daily for forty days

   Maintenance Protocol

   - Liposomal NAD+ or NAD+ Precursors: Niacinamide, NMN, or NR
   - Supporting Compounds: Urolithin A, Resveratrol, PQQ, Quercetin, Apigenin

6. **Stress Management**
   - Positive Mindset: Visualize your healthiest self
   - Adaptogenic Support (add as needed):
     - L-theanine
     - Rhodiola Rosea
     - Ashwagandha
     - Relora
     - Selank (available as a nasal spray)—particularly beneficial for anxiety

7. **Immunomodulation Support**
   - Low-Dose Naltrexone (LDN)
   - TB4 Fragment
   - Thymogen Alpha 1

8. **Gut-Healing Protocol**
    - Therapeutic Agents: Nitazoxanide/larazotide (especially if the TMAO level is high)
    - Healing Support: BPC-157 (provides systemic healing in addition to gut healing)
    - Microbiome Support:
        - Prebiotic: Inulin powder (or other broad-spectrum, diverse fiber blend such as Fiber MGP from OrthoMolecular)
        - Probiotic: Spore-based formulations or better yet, fermented vegetables such as sour kraut/kimchi/real pickles
        - Postbiotic: Tributyrin

General Peptide Classification

The following is a general peptide classification by location and primary activity.

Immune-Modulating Peptides

(Thymus gland-related) and gut-brain axis peptides

Thymosin beta
TB4 Frag (oral)
Thymosin Alpha 1
Thymogen Alpha 1 (oral)
BPC 157 (oral)
KPV (oral)
TB4 Active Frag
Zn-thymulin
Delta Sleep-Inducing Peptide (DSIP)
GHK-Cu
Cerebrolysin
CerebroPep (oral)

Pineal Gland Peptides

modulate thymus, lengthen telomeres, modulate immunity, sleep, and the hypothalamic-pituitary-hormone axes

Epitalon
Pinealon
Delta sleep-inducing peptide (DSIP)
Testagen
Melatonin

Gastrointestinal/Leaky Gut/Inflammatory Bowel Disease/ Gut-Brain Axis Peptides

BPC-15
TB4 Active Frag
KPV
Delta sleep-inducing peptide (DSIP)
GHK-Cu
LL-37
Tuftin
Livagen
Larazotide (Zonulin antagonist)

Brain Peptides

Cerebrolysin (IV)/CerebroPep (oral)
Semax
Selank
BPC 157
TB4 Active Frag
DSIP
KPV
Humanin
SS-31
MOTSc
5 Amino 1 MQ
GHK-Cu
PE 22-28
P21
Methylene Blue
ARA-290
Cortexin
Dihexa

Antimicrobial Peptides

LL-37
BPC 157
TB4/Active Frag
KPV
GHK-Cu
Methylene Blue

Mitochondrial Peptides

MOTSc
SS 31
Humanin
SLU PP 332
5 amino 1 MQ
BPC 157
TB4 Active Frag
Small human-like peptides
DSIP
T3 (liothyronine)
Melatonin
PQQ
Methylene Blue
mitoquinone
ubiquinol

Rejuvenation/Pain/Anabolic/Healing Peptides

BPC 157
TB4/TB4 Active Frag
Vilon
Epitalon
Pinealon
DSIP
AOD 9604 (fragment of HGH)
GHC-Cu
KPV
Cerebrolysin (IV)
CerebroPep (oral)
FOX 04-DRI
Follistatin
ACE-031
ARA 290
Cardiogen
Carnosine

GHRH/GHRP

Growth hormone-releasing hormones and growth hormone-releasing peptides—stimulate growth hormone production and secretion

Sermorelin CJC 1295, tesamorelin, hexarelin, ibutamoren (MK-677), ipamorelin

Sleep/Anti-Anxiety Peptides

DSIP
Epitalon
Pinealon
Growth hormone (using GHRH/GHRPs)
AOD
Selank
BPC 157
KPV

Building a Personalized Wellness Strategy

One-size-fits-all wellness approaches simply don't deliver as advertised. Biological pathways, genetic predispositions, and lifestyle factors that determine individual wellness trajectories are as unique as fingerprints. What works remarkably well for one person may prove ineffective or even counterproductive for another, highlighting the critical importance of personalized strategies in achieving optimal health outcomes. Fortunately, modern wellness is seeing the rise of a new paradigm of precision health optimization.

Modern wellness optimization begins with understanding the intricate interplay between our genetic blueprint, environmental influences, and lifestyle choices. Today's advanced genetic testing allows us to identify specific variants that affect everything from nutrient metabolism and exercise response to stress resilience and sleep patterns. When combined with comprehensive lifestyle assessments and biomarker analysis, such testing creates a detailed map of individual health needs and vulnerabilities.

I believe that traditional wellness protocols often overlook the fundamental reality that our bodies operate as highly individualized biological systems. For example, a Mediterranean diet might be transformative for someone with specific genetic variants related to fat metabolism while proving less beneficial for another individual whose genetic profile suggests better outcomes with alternative nutritional approaches. Similarly, high-intensity interval training may optimize cardiovascular health for one person while potentially increasing cortisol burden in another with different stress response genetics.

One particularly powerful solution is the integration of peptide therapy into personalized wellness, representing a sophisticated advancement in whole-being health. These naturally occurring biological messengers can be strategically selected and administered based on individual needs, genetic predispositions, and specific health goals. This personalized approach extends beyond supplementation to encompass lifestyle modifications, exercise programming, and stress management techniques tailored to individual characteristics. By understanding how our genes influence our response to various interventions, we can make more informed decisions about nutrition timing, exercise selection, sleep optimization, and stress-reduction strategies that align with our biological predispositions rather than working against them.

Indeed, peptides can be used to target specific areas of health optimization, such as improving skin elasticity, reducing inflammation, enhancing cognitive function, or boosting muscle recovery. How does this work?

Key Peptides for Muscle Recovery

Let's focus on muscle recovery as an illustration. When it comes to optimizing muscle recovery through peptide therapy, several compounds stand out for their targeted benefits. These peptides work through different mechanisms to enhance healing, reduce inflammation, and accelerate the recovery process.

Epitalon: The Sleep-Recovery Connection

Epitalon serves as a foundational peptide for muscle recovery by significantly improving sleep quality. It enhances both deep sleep and REM sleep phases—the most restorative periods with peak muscle repair and growth hormone release. This improved sleep architecture translates directly into enhanced recovery capacity.

What makes this particularly valuable is that we can now measure these improvements objectively. Today's popular, wearable technology, like smartwatches and recovery rings, provides baseline data, allowing you to track your recovery scores before and after implementing Epitalon therapy.

BPC-157

We discussed earlier in the book that BPC-157 earned its nickname as the "Wolverine peptide" due to its remarkable healing properties. This compound directly targets muscle recovery by:

- Reducing inflammation at the injury site
- Accelerating tissue repair and regeneration
- Promoting blood vessel formation to improve nutrient delivery
- Supporting connective tissue healing

TB-4 Fragment: Immune-Enhanced Recovery

TB-4 fragment, derived from thymus gland peptides, offers a dual approach to muscle recovery. Beyond its direct healing properties, it provides immune modulation benefits that support the body's natural recovery processes. This peptide promotes neurogenesis and enhances spatial memory while delivering neuroprotective and neuro-restorative effects.

Stacking for Maximum Benefits

The real power of peptide therapy for muscle recovery lies in strategic stacking. Rather than relying on a single compound, combining these peptides creates synergistic effects such as:

- Epitalon for sleep optimization and foundational recovery
- BPC-157 for direct tissue healing and inflammation reduction
- TB-4 fragment for immune support and additional healing enhancement

This combination addresses multiple aspects of the recovery process simultaneously, potentially delivering superior results compared to any single peptide alone.

Let's look at a real-time chronology of peptide therapy administered within our health center, a multimodal approach to health optimization in a high-performance aging athlete. As you will see, if we are comprehensive with our approach and hit it from every angle, we can see significant improvements. And that's the case with this patient, a professional car racer. He has been extremely dedicated and motivated to do all the right things and is doing very, very well with his events, even being decades older than his competitors.

Case Study

PATIENT PROFILE

Age: 67-year-old male

Occupation/Background: Former collegiate and professional Major League Baseball player; current high-performance race car driver (GT World Challenge America); member of the Seven Summits Club at Snowbird, Utah.

Clinical Summary

DP is a 67-year-old active male with a remarkable history of lifelong athleticism and competitive performance. He is a long-standing concierge patient and a personal friend, having once been my college roommate. Over the past decade, DP has been fully engaged in a comprehensive, integrative health optimization program that mirrors my own clinical and personal regimen, tailored to his unique medical and performance needs.

Despite his age, DP remains highly competitive in the GT World Challenge America racing circuit, often outperforming competitors decades younger. He attributes his sustained success to his dedication to a highly structured, multifactorial health regimen, supported by functional medicine principles.

MEDICAL HISTORY

Chronic Conditions

- Hyperlipidemia, including elevated lipoprotein(a)
- Stage 2 chronic kidney disease (likely NSAID-induced)
- Chronic inflammatory response syndrome (CIRS)
- Degenerative disc disease (cervical and lumbar)
- Chronic neck and low back pain

- Migraine headaches
- Prediabetes
- Elevated homocysteine due to MTHFR polymorphism

Surgeries/Procedures

- Total shoulder replacement
- Multiple orthopedic interventions due to prior sports injuries and car racing incidents

Medication History

- Chronic use of Celebrex
- Intermittent use of Percocet
- Long-term use of Ambien and Trazodone for sleep

Initial Presenting Complaints (circa 7–8 years ago)

- Suboptimal sleep (poor deep and REM phases)
- Chronic musculoskeletal pain
- Inflammatory burden (as evidenced by biomarkers and symptomology)
- Poor recovery capacity post-exercise or exertion
- Mild weight gain with associated loss of lean mass and endurance

Comprehensive Functional and Regenerative Medicine Intervention

DP's regimen reflects an aggressive, full-spectrum approach to systemic inflammation, age-related degeneration, and performance optimization.

Pharmaceutical and Peptide-Based Interventions:

- Low-Dose Naltrexone (LDN) for immunomodulation
- Losartan for inflammation and TGF-β1 modulation
- Testosterone undecanoate injections (every 8 weeks)
- CJC-1295 with Ipamorelin for GH support
- Oral peptides (AM and PM):
    - TB4 Frag
    - Thymogen Alpha-1
    - BPC-157
    - KPV
    - Epitalon

Regenerative Interventions

- Multiple rounds of **mesenchymal stem cell therapy**, including:
  - **Intravenous stem cell infusions** for systemic and neurological support
  - **Localized musculoskeletal injections** for joint and soft tissue recovery
- **Exosome therapy** administered in parallel with stem cells to enhance intercellular signaling and regenerative outcomes

Nutraceuticals and Supplements (non-exhaustive, highlights below):

Anti-Inflammatory & Metabolic

- Berberine
- Slow-release niacin
- Methylated B-complex (for MTHFR)
- N-acetylcysteine (for liver and oxidative stress)
- 7-Keto DHEA
- Pro-resolving mediators (SPMs)
- Ubiquinol

Mitochondrial and Cognitive Support

- Mitocore mitochondrial multivitamin
- Urolithin A, Resveratrol, PQQ, NAD+ precursors
- Liposomal NAD+

GI Health and Detoxification

- General probiotic
- Spore-based probiotic with immunoglobulins
- Digestive enzymes with meals
- Tributyrin
- TUDCA

Musculoskeletal and Joint Health

- Creatine 5–15g daily
- Collagen-rich phospholipid blend on days he's not eating eggs

- Joint complex (SynovX DJD)
- Topical GHK-Cu cream

Cardiovascular Support

- Bergamot (1000 mg daily)
- Fish oil (EPA + DHA = 1640mg/day)
- Fiber/prebiotic supplements

Other Interventions

- Hair, skin, nails complex
- Shilajit blend
- Lysine 1000 mg/day
- Thyroid support formula
- Regular endurance and strength training

OUTCOMES AND PROGRESS

Within 12–18 months of initiating the program:

Pain Management: No more reliance on Celebrex and discontinuation of Percocet

Sleep: Improved architecture, eliminated use of Ambien and Trazodone

Body Composition: Lean mass preserved or improved; body fat reduced

Performance: Enhanced recovery, stamina, and strength; notable endurance improvements

Labs: normalization of renal function markers, reduction in inflammatory markers (e.g., TGF-β1, CRP cardiac), improved homocysteine levels with methylation support

Post-Stem Cell Therapy: Subjectively improved recovery, pain reduction, and overall vitality within weeks of IV stem cell + exosome therapy

DISCUSSION

DP's success reflects the synergy between commitment, personalization, regenerative medicine, and data-driven strategy in long-term health optimization. His protocol attacks inflammation, mitochondrial decline, hormonal imbalance, and musculoskeletal degeneration through a combination of traditional functional medicine and advanced regenerative therapies.

Notably, DP underwent multiple rounds of mesenchymal stem cell and exosome therapy, both intravenously and intra-articularly. These treatments likely contributed to the marked improvements in pain, recovery time, vitality, and joint integrity, particularly given his orthopedic and degenerative spine history. He is very convinced that the oral peptides also drastically improved his outcomes.

This case exemplifies the potential of personalized, systems-based medicine—especially when the patient is motivated, consistent, and resourced. As I've told DP many times, my role is to map the strategy, but it's up to him to "drive the race." His results speak to the power of disciplined compliance and a holistic approach to anti-aging and performance optimization.

CONCLUSION

DP remains a thriving example of what's possible when a patient fully commits to the principles of functional and regenerative medicine. With unwavering dedication and a willingness to explore cutting-edge therapies, he has not only avoided decline but has actually improved in multiple domains—athletic, cognitive, metabolic, and emotional—despite being in his late sixties.

Today, DP continues to race competitively, ski aggressively, and serve his family and community from a place of strength, clarity, and health. His journey is a testament to the power of comprehensive, multifaceted health optimization.

Peptide Benefits for Skin Health and Cognitive Function

In addition to muscle recovery, skin health and cognitive processes are also common patient concerns. Let's take a closer look at the role of peptides in these areas.

Skin Health and Anti-Aging Benefits

Several peptides offer significant benefits for skin health and elasticity. When we achieve better restorative sleep patterns through peptide supplementation, our bodies heal more effectively, leading to positive effects on connective tissue repair and overall skin health.

Comprehensive Anti-Aging Benefits

Epitalon stands out as particularly effective in this area. A bioregulatory peptide, Epitalon contains extensive anti-aging properties:

Cellular Health

- Lengthens telomeres and slows aging processes
- Decreases mortality and increases life expectancy
- Normalizes antioxidant pathways and reduces oxidative stress

Sleep and Circadian Function

- Improves pineal gland function
- Normalizes circadian rhythms and melatonin production
- Enhances deep sleep and REM sleep quality

Metabolic and Cardiovascular Benefits

- Improves insulin sensitivity
- Decreases LDL ("bad") cholesterol
- Raises HDL ("good") cholesterol
- Enhances tissue repair throughout the body

Epitalon also gets "bonus points" for boosting immunity through improved thymus function, demonstrating anti-cancer activity, and improving sex hormone regulation.

BPC-157 also provides notable skin benefits through its healing properties. Another important peptide for skin health is **GHK-Cu**, a copper peptide that significantly increases collagen production. This peptide is commonly found in topical skincare formulations and creams. While it can be taken orally, it requires a liposomal (fat-soluble) form to achieve optimal absorption and effectiveness when consumed rather than applied topically.

Cognitive Function Enhancement

Several peptides show promise for cognitive improvement.

BPC-157 has demonstrated remarkable healing properties that extend to brain tissue and the blood-brain barrier. Research shows it can:

- Counteract cognitive dysfunction
- Reduce social withdrawal and anhedonia
- Influence neurotransmitter systems involved in cognition
- Provide neuroprotection through multiple pathways, including reduced oxidative stress and increased neurogenic differentiation

Of special note, the cognitive benefits of BPC-157 make sense given its role in promoting quality restorative sleep, which directly impacts cognitive function.

Specialized Cognitive Peptides

DIHEXA shows significant brain-enhancing effects and has demonstrated therapeutic potential in neurodegenerative conditions like Parkinson's disease.

Cerebrolysin consists of brain-derived peptides from porcine sources and promotes neuro-regeneration. While traditional Cerebrolysin requires injection, an oral equivalent called **Cerebral Pep** (made by Integrative Peptides) provides similar benefits.

TB-4 Fragment offers multiple neurological benefits:

- Promotes neurogenesis (creation of new brain cells)
- Enhances spatial memory
- Shows positive effects in Alzheimer's disease research
- Provides neuroprotective and neuro-restorative properties

Methylene Blue: Mitochondrial Enhancement

While not technically a peptide, methylene blue deserves mention as a popular cognitive supplement. It provides pronounced mitochondrial enhancement benefits, and since improved mitochondrial function directly correlates with better cognitive performance, users typically notice cognitive improvements relatively quickly.

All told, the interconnected nature of these benefits becomes clear when considering how improved sleep quality, enhanced cellular repair, and optimized mitochondrial function all contribute to better overall health. In the chapter to come, we'll optimize the Big Five foundational principles from Part Two, from a treatment perspective, on the path to vibrant, long-lasting health.

CHAPTER 12

Optimizing Your Biological Blueprint

Epigenetics (how genes express themselves) shows us that we are not prisoners of our DNA, but authors of our health.

Functional Medicine axiom

Your DNA is your blueprint, but epigenetics determine how that blueprint is read and implemented—and it is profoundly influenced by lifestyle, environment, nutrition, stress, toxins, and even your thoughts and emotions.

The human body operates through the inner workings of five interconnected biological systems (i.e., the Big Five), each requiring precision-targeted interventions for all individuals. But traditional wellness treats these biological systems as separate entities, ignoring their interconnectedness. Understanding how your genetic blueprint influences the Big Five creates the foundation for transformative health outcomes based on genetic predispositions and lifestyle factors.

To fully understand the intricate web of wellness, we must first realize how one system's strand's activity amplifies the impact on another, and another after that. But a fundamental flaw in traditional treatment protocols is a reductionist approach to our bodies' interconnected biological ecosystems. One needs only to look to nature to see the importance and seamless operation of everything in sync. A forest cannot thrive on soil alone, while ignoring water sources, sunlight, and symbiotic relationships between species. In similar fashion, optimal human health cannot be achieved by targeting isolated systems while neglecting their intricate interdependencies.

The gut microbiome communicates directly with brain function through the gut-brain axis, while mitochondrial energy production affects immune system capacity (and in reality, every cell in the body), which in turn influences stress resilience and spiritual well-being. This interconnected reality demands a comprehensive assessment approach that leaves no biological stone unturned. Over years of clinical practice, I've discovered that sustainable health optimization requires simultaneous attention to all five foundational pillars, with specific interventions and testing protocols strategically simplified based on an individual's presentation patterns.

Optimal human health cannot be achieved by targeting isolated systems while neglecting their intricate interdependencies.

This ecosystem principle applies at every level—from cellular communication networks to organ system interactions to broader environmental influences shaping our biological responses. Honoring these connections, rather than fragmenting them, unlocks the body's remarkable capacity for systemic healing and optimization. And if we don't look under every stone, we could find (or not find) things that can slow optimal health progress and success.

I've done my best over the years to simplify assessment approaches that can provide necessary information without excessive testing. The key lies in understanding which diagnostic approaches yield the most actionable insights for an individual's unique biological landscape.

Let's first look at a high-level view of clinical acumen gleaned over my nearly forty years of practicing functional medicine.

Assessment Methods

Strategic simplification often yields the most actionable insight, and I've learned and implemented those diagnostic approaches that provide essential information without excessive complexity or cost. For example, my approach to gastrointestinal evaluation has evolved significantly over the years. In the past, I did a lot of SIBO (small intestinal bacterial overgrowth) testing. In fact, I operated the first SIBO breath-testing machine in Utah and utilized this technology extensively for decades. But my current protocols, along with the integration of peptide therapies, have allowed me to achieve comparable therapeutic outcomes through more streamlined assessment methods.

Today I rely primarily on specific blood markers that accurately reflect intestinal permeability, including the MMP-9 test as a reliable indicator of gut barrier function, while TMAO levels provide additional insight into intestinal health status. These markers effectively guide treatment protocols without the complexity and expense of breath testing or comprehensive stool analysis with microbiome mapping (though I do reserve these advanced diagnostics for cases that don't respond to initial therapeutic approaches).

Food Sensitivity Testing

Another interesting arena is food sensitivity testing. Early in my career, I routinely ordered comprehensive IgG food sensitivity panels covering dozens of potential allergens. However, most food sensitivities are secondary manifestations of gut dysfunction rather than primary immune reactions. Healing the gut typically resolves the majority of these sensitivities naturally. I now focus on two key markers: IgG gluten sensitivity and IgG candida antibody levels. (Gluten is an exception to the secondary sensitivity principle, as genetic predisposition affects a significant portion of the population.) Additionally, most American gluten-containing products are tainted with glyphosate (an herbicide!), which creates an inflammatory burden that damages gut integrity regardless of genetic sensitivity.

That said, my food sensitivity testing also includes candida antibody assessment that provides insight into yeast overgrowth patterns without requiring comprehensive fungal culture testing. I specifically utilize IgG antibodies rather than IgM, as these represent the immune system's longer-term memory response and provide more clinically relevant information for chronic conditions.

Immune System Evaluation

Moving on to immune system evaluation, I simplify testing here as well, focusing inflammation assessment on C-reactive protein, specifically the cardiac-selective variant, which gives me an idea of the degree of arterial and endothelial inflammatory activity. I include erythrocyte sedimentation rate (ESR) when systemic autoimmune conditions like rheumatoid arthritis or lupus are suspected.

While comprehensive cytokine panels through LabCorp can evaluate TH1 and TH2 immune balance, I've found these unnecessary for most treatment decisions. Similarly, natural killer cell activity testing, though valuable for chronic inflammatory response syndrome (CIRS) evaluation, rarely influences my therapeutic approach when combined with symptom assessment and other available markers.

A WORD ON NATURAL KILLER CELLS

These cells function as the immune system's frontline defense, targeting pathogenic microbes and foreign organisms that don't belong in the body. In CIRS, a characteristic immune dysregulation develops where the TH1 pathway becomes progressively underactive as the condition becomes more chronic. Simultaneously, the TH2 pathway becomes overactive.

This fundamental immune imbalance creates the hallmark dysfunction seen in CIRS patients. While natural killer cell activity testing can provide insight into this dysregulation, I've discovered that transforming growth factor beta-1 levels offer the most clinically useful information for assessing immune imbalance severity and treatment progress.

My commitment to diagnostic simplification has allowed me to significantly streamline these assessments. Many physicians following traditional CIRS protocols, such as the original Shoemaker approach, routinely order extensive testing batteries, but years of clinical experience have taught me that most of these tests prove unnecessary for effective treatment planning and monitoring.

For CIRS cases specifically, transforming growth factor beta-1 levels provide the most clinically useful information about immune imbalance between the T-regulatory and TH17 pathways. This single marker often eliminates the need for extensive testing protocols traditionally associated with biotoxin illness treatment.

Autoimmune and Mitochondrial Screening

Moving from autoimmune through mitochondrial function, I screen every new patient for Hashimoto's thyroiditis due to its prevalence and significant impact on overall health optimization. Additional autoimmune panels are individualized based on clinical presentation and family history rather than applied universally. Neurotransmitter metabolite testing rarely provides actionable information in my current practice. Interestingly, heart rate variability (HRV) assessment, once requiring specialized equipment, is now accessible through consumer devices like smartwatches and Oura rings. Patients can track their autonomic nervous system balance at home continuously during treatment, providing real-time feedback on therapeutic progress.

Direct mitochondrial function testing remains challenging, though emerging technologies from European laboratories show promise. Currently, I assess mitochondrial health through clinical history combined with metabolic markers. For instance, the insulin resistance score from advanced lipid profiling (utilizing NMR(MRI)-based particle size analysis) correlates well with mitochondrial dysfunction. Traditional markers like fasting glucose, fasting insulin, and calculated ratios (HOMA-IR—homeostasis model assessment of insulin resistance) provide additional insight into cellular energy metabolism.

All told, VO2 max testing represents the gold standard for mitochondrial assessment, though practical limitations make this impractical for routine use. Clinical evaluation of energy levels, exercise tolerance, and recovery patterns typically provides sufficient information for treatment planning. In America, an estimated 94 percent have at least some degree of mitochondrial dysfunction. We all have work to do!

Over years of clinical observation, I've realized (and experienced firsthand) that optimal health requires addressing all interconnected systems, but diagnostic complexity doesn't necessarily improve therapeutic outcomes. By focusing on the most informative tests for each biological system, we can develop comprehensive treatment strategies while maintaining practical efficiency and cost-effectiveness.

The key lies in understanding which assessments provide actionable intelligence versus academic interest, allowing us to honor the body's interconnected nature while avoiding diagnostic paralysis.

Integrated Treatment Protocols for Comprehensive Health Optimization

Below are details of targeted protocols we employ in our practice's optimal health plans.

Assessment and Baseline Establishment

Comprehensive Testing Matrix

Baseline Functional Panel

- Cbc
- Cmp 20 including an uric acid level
- Lipoprofile NMR with an insulin resistance score

- Apolipoprotein B
    - HOMA calculation
    - Ferritin
- CRP cardiac
- Fibrinogen antigen
    - Homocysteine status (critical to optimize before detoxification)
- Hormone panel to include:

  tsh, free T4, free T3, reverse T3, IGF-1, total and free testosterone, dhea sulfate, ACTH, morning cortisol, estradiol, progesterone (for women), LH and FSH (if indicated), ADH, Melanocyte-stimulating hormone, fasting insulin, and fasting leptin (if indicated)

Gut Function Panel

- MMP9 (matrix metalloproteinase 9)
- TMAO (trimethylamine N-oxide)

  when needed:

    - Comprehensive stool analysis with microbiome mapping
    - Intestinal permeability assessment
    - SIBO/SIFO breath testing
    - Food sensitivity and IgG panels

Immune System Evaluation

- TGFB1 (transforming growth factor beta 1)
- HNK1 (CD57 count)—if chronic Lyme disease (with or without coinfections) is suspected

  when indicated, the following:

    - Complete inflammatory marker panel (CRP, ESR, cytokines)
    - Consider TH1/TH2 cytokine panel with LabCorp

- Natural killer cell activity
- Immunoglobulin levels and subclasses
- Autoimmune screening battery (at least include a TPO -thyroid peroxidase)

Neurological Assessment (when indicated, the following)

- HRV and autonomic nervous system testing—smart watch/Oura ring tracking
- Cognitive function baseline testing
- Sleep study and circadian rhythm markers—tracking with smart watch/Oura ring

Mitochondrial Function Testing

- Organic acids test (OAT)
- VO2 max testing if able
- ATP production capacity
- Oxidative stress markers
- Nutrient cofactor status (such as Coenzyme Q10 levels)
- Metabolomics testing

Spiritual/Emotional Baseline

- Stress assessment questionnaires/history taking
- Life purpose and meaning inventories
- Social connection and support mapping

Foundation Building

Gut Restoration Protocol

Remove and Reset

- Anti-inflammatory/autoimmune diet—when indicated, start with a low-lectin, gut-healing diet such as

Dr. Gundry's "Plant Paradox" and graduate to a modified paleo diet (allowing for A2 casein dairy for most patients)
- Digestive enzyme support
- Stress reduction initiation

Repair and Restore

- L-glutamine and gut lining nutrients (when indicated)
- Immunoglobulin supplementation such as colostrum
- Consider nitazoxanide/larazotide compounded prescription if the TMAO level is elevated—typically for one month then pulse treatment—one out of every four weeks for four months
- BPC 157
- Targeted probiotic introduction—at least a spore-based probiotic, or better yet, fermented veggies
- Prebiotic fiber gradual increase
- Vagus nerve stimulation practices (consider external vagal nerve stimulator use)

Re-inoculate and Maintain

- Diverse probiotic rotation
- Fermented food integration
- Postbiotic supplementation—Tributyrin for 2 months

Simultaneous Interventions

Mitochondrial Support Initiation

- Methylene Blue 4–16 mg/day in the morning
- Omega-3—marine based—maintenance EPA + DHA = 1,500–2,000mg but consider doubling that to "load" for two months or so (consider OmegaQuant testing baseline and after a few months of use to ascertain optimal levels)

- Vitamin D3/K2 (measure and treat)—Remember that the sun is our friend. Avoid burning but get some color and keep it. It will serve you well.
- Magnesium optimization
- B-vitamin complex with active forms (methylated Bs—more aggressive dosing for higher homocysteine levels)
- Mitochondrial supporting multivitamin with methylated Bs, alpha lipoic acid, chromium, acetyl L-carnitine, biotin, zinc, selenium, resveratrol, and more
- Coenzyme Q10 or ubiquinol for those over fifty years or age
- PQQ
- Low-carb or even a healthy version of a ketogenic diet
- Intermittent fasting

Red Light Therapy

- Basic Immune Modulation—supplements covered in "Mitochondrial Support Initiation"
    - Omega-3 fatty acids (EPA/DHA)
    - Vitamin D3 optimization
    - Zinc and selenium support

Spiritual Practice Introduction

- Daily meditation (at least ten to fifteen minutes)
- Gratitude journaling—perhaps most important of all!
- Nature connection time

Section 1: Advanced Optimization and Enhancement

Advanced Gut-Brain Axis Support

- Reassess digestive symptoms and retest gut inflammatory markers such as TMAO and MMP9
    - Continue an anti-inflammatory diet, allowing for occasional "smart indiscretions"

- Vagal Tone Enhancement
    - Cold exposure therapy—stimulates the sympathetic followed by the parasympathetic sides of the ANS (autonomic nervous system)
    - Breathing exercises (box breathing, Wim Hof)
    - Singing/humming practices
    - Grounding—ideally barefoot on the ground—with nature
- Vagal nerve stimulator use (external)

Immune System Fine-Tuning

- Advanced Anti-Inflammatory Protocol
    - Liposomal curcumin
    - Specialized pro-resolving mediators (SPMs)—especially if still inflamed/in pain
- Immune Training
    - Controlled hormetic stressors including consideration of HBOT (hyperbaric oxygen therapy)
    - Sauna therapy protocols
    - Intermittent fasting windows
- Consider LDN (low-dose naltrexone), Thymogen Alpha 1, and TB4 Frag when indicated

Mitochondrial Enhancement

NAD+ Optimization

- NAD+ IV therapy if able to commit to the time and cost
- Or NAD+ subcutaneous injections
- Liposomal NAD+ orally
- In some cases, may need to consider first treating one month with five amino 1 mq
- Urolithin A to enhance mitophagy
- PQQ, quercetin/apigenin

- Red light therapy
- AMPK activation strategies such as with Rapamycin

Neurological Optimization

Neurotransmitter Support (if indicated)

- Tyrosine for dopamine
- 5-HTP for serotonin (if indicated)
- GABA support (theanine, taurine)

Cognitive Enhancement

- Never forget methylene blue consideration
- Bacopa monnieri (blunts the stress/cortisol response)
- Lion's Mane mushroom
- Ashwagandha
- Rhodiola rosea
- BPC 157 peptide
- Cerebrolysin or orally CerebroPep peptide
- Dihexa peptide
- Don't forget parasympathetic tone considerations

Spiritual and Emotional Integration

Advanced Practices

- Extended meditation sessions—focusing on gratitude
- Breathwork intensives
- Service-oriented activities
- Creative expression cultivation

Advanced Integration and Personalization

Personalized Protocol Refinement

Genetic Considerations

- MTHFR and methylation support—make sure the homocysteine level is measured and optimized early on in the process
- APOE4 and neuroprotection—consider studying/following Dr. Dale Bredesen's work on reversing dementia
- COMT and dopamine metabolism—as indicated

Advanced Testing and Adjustment

- Repeat comprehensive panels—at least repeat the abnormal tests that we are optimizing
- Protocol modification based on progress
- Biomarker-driven fine-tuning

Advanced Interventions

Cutting-Edge Modalities

- Red light therapy protocols
- Hyperbaric oxygen therapy
- Neurofeedback training
- IV nutrient therapy consideration
- IV autologous hemotransfusion with ozone and UV light
- If indicated at this point—accurate testing for chronic infections such as chronic Lyme disease, coinfections, chronic viral infections, and others
- Consider SOT (selective oligonucleotide therapy) if indicated (the hope is that by treating foundationally and immunomodulating that we can avoid the need for these more advanced and more expensive therapies)

- Note: "it's the terrain not the germ"—optimize the terrain (gut/immune/neurologic/mitochondrial) first and the terrain will hopefully "take care of" the germ

---

Section 2: Maintenance and Long-Term Optimization

Sustainable Lifestyle Integration

80/20 Rule Application

- Core non-negotiables
- Flexible adaptation strategies—once health is optimized, we should be able to "tolerate" smart indiscretions periodically without setbacks
- Social and travel considerations—I pack my stacks and travel with them personally

Monitoring and Adjustment Protocols

Regular Assessment Schedule

- Quarterly biomarker reviews
- Annual comprehensive testing
- Subjective wellness tracking

Advanced Troubleshooting

Plateau-Breaking Strategies

- Protocol cycling approaches
- Novel intervention integration
- Stress and life change adaptations

Section 3: Special Considerations and Contraindications

Individual Variations

- Age-specific modifications
- Gender-based considerations
- Genetic polymorphism adaptations
- Chronic condition modifications

Safety Protocols

- Supplement interactions
- Medical supervision requirements
- Red flag symptoms
- When to seek professional help

The Integrated Wellness Paradigm

- Viewing health as an emergent property of system interactions
- The importance of patience and consistency
- Building resilience for long-term wellness
- Evolution and adaptation of protocols over time

If the desire and vision are there to begin with, and we commit and stay the course with patience and consistency, we can and will improve our health. We can all optimize our health with this approach.

Optimizing for Resilience

I believe foundational health emerges not from isolated interventions but from the dynamic interplay between interconnected biological systems. As soil grows a tree that affects wildlife that in turn impacts nutrient cycling, our bodies function similarly. Our bodies are integrated networks where gut health influences brain function, mitochondrial energy production affects immune capacity, and spiritual well-being shapes stress resilience.

This systems-based understanding demands a fundamental shift in how we approach wellness optimization. Rather than seeking quick fixes or targeting isolated symptoms, sustainable health improvement requires patience and unwavering consistency. Biological adaptations that create lasting vitality occur gradually, often imperceptibly, as cellular repair mechanisms, metabolic pathways, and immune responses recalibrate.

Building resilience becomes the cornerstone of long-term wellness success. Resilient biological systems can adapt to stressors, recover from setbacks, and maintain optimal function despite environmental challenges. This resilience develops through consistent application of personalized protocols. Perhaps most importantly, effective wellness optimization requires evolutionary thinking. Protocols must adapt as our bodies change, as new research emerges, and as life circumstances shift. The approaches that optimize health at age thirty may require refinement at age fifty. The interventions that work during periods of low stress may need adjustment during stressful life transitions to ensure continued progress.

Remember that the path to optimal health demands vision and commitment. Those who approach wellness optimization with a clear intention, realistic expectations, and dedication to consistency will experience profound improvements in energy, cognitive function, emotional resilience, and overall vitality. This integrated approach, rooted in biological reality rather than marketing promises, offers genuine hope for transformative health outcomes.

The human body possesses remarkable capacity for healing and optimization when provided with the right conditions, interventions, and time to respond. By honoring the interconnected nature of our biological systems and maintaining consistency with personalized protocols, we can all achieve the levels of health and vitality we wish to achieve. From there, we are poised to move beyond a baseline understanding and take practical steps toward integrating these practices into daily life.

CHAPTER 13

Empowering a Healthy Life

The best way to predict the future is to create it.

Abraham Lincoln

Consider for a moment the pursuit of professional fulfillment, an exhilarating, frustrating, interminable quest in which we often liken career success with life satisfaction. But what does satisfaction mean to you? Professional achievements can offer temporary satisfaction, but genuine well-being blooms from aligning our daily choices with what truly matters to us. I believe the path to fulfillment and contentment lies in curating a lifestyle that resonates with our deepest values and aspirations.

This perspective opens the door to sustainable health and authentic success measured not by external metrics but by the quality of life we create for ourselves. And it starts by making informed decisions that will best benefit your health. When it comes to peptide therapy, seeking guidance from the right kind of provider is critical. Many of my recommendations, particularly for the peptides discussed in this book, depend largely on blood test results. While we don't necessarily need to be overly concerned about safety issues without blood tests, we will certainly be more accurately guided toward optimal health when working with someone who can guide and periodically monitor progress.

The unfortunate reality is that there aren't many providers, or even functional medicine practitioners, who are well-versed enough in adding peptides to treatment regimens (a somewhat new, unique, and specialized expertise).

Finding the Right Guide

So what exactly is a functional medicine specialist as opposed to a traditional general practice physician? In a basic definition, functional medicine providers can include medical doctors, doctors of osteopathy, naturopathic physicians, some chiropractors, nurse practitioners, or physician assistants. They might even be practitioners who specialize in functional medicine within the nutritional realm. Some personal trainers are even well-versed enough in this area to help guide people effectively. Overall, the field is fairly broad in terms of credentials.

What sets functional medicine providers apart is their focus on finding and treating *root causes* of illness rather than just managing symptoms. While there are quite a few functional medicine providers who claim this approach, which is great, what we are outlining here goes one step beyond that standard to optimize health—to reach the next level of wellness. This represents a more advanced approach than what people might typically receive from traditional functional medicine. We're talking about providers that not only follow functional medicine principles where they focus on root causes but also integrate strategies that go beyond to truly optimize health.

That said, when searching for a provider, the key is connecting with someone who is equipped with peptide-specific experience and knowledge. You want to ensure they understand what they're dealing with and can provide advice that delivers the most benefit to your health journey.

Ensuring Quality

Next up on the well-being empowerment checklist is understanding product quality, an absolutely crucial step. Peptides are incredibly popular right now—a hot topic with significant hype surrounding them—and unfortunately, this has inspired many substandard products to flood the market. The best way to navigate this? Lean on the old "if it's too good to be true, it probably is" adage. If you find a less expensive peptide product, there is typically a reason it's cheaper.

Do your homework to ensure you're getting a reputable product that has been third-party tested and continues to be third-party tested—not just testing one batch, but sourcing from companies that continually retest their products for quality and purity.

Currently, most oral peptides operate in an unregulated space and are easily found online. However, there are fewer than half a dozen brands that I would have any confidence in recommending (our Haven brand being one of them, of course).

Oral vs. Injection: Understanding Your Options

One question I commonly hear is whether these peptides work orally and whether they are better injected versus taken orally. The orally available peptides we've discussed in this book, particularly those for treating inflammation and supporting various bodily functions, do work effectively when taken orally—provided it's a high-quality product that is properly formulated with enteric coating and capped ends.

However, there is an important point to keep in mind. All of the peptides we've covered, with the exception of BPC-157, are remarkably short (four amino acids in length or shorter). Some contain only two amino acids (called dipeptides), while others contain three (tripeptides), and still others contain four (tetrapeptides). We often refer to these short amino acid chains as bioregulatory peptides or bioregulators.

Because these peptides are so short, it is much less likely that they will be digested into individual amino acids before absorption and utilization. Instead, they are quickly and easily absorbed into the bloodstream, especially when formulated properly with protective caps. Once absorbed, they effectively send their inherent signals and mimic well what the body naturally produces—though in many cases, the body isn't producing them in sufficient quantities.

As a side note, BPC-157 presents an interesting case. While it is a longer amino acid chain (fifteen amino acids in length), it is naturally produced in the stomach's gastric juices. Because of this, the body recognizes it as something that shouldn't simply be digested away. Again, provided it's a high-quality, properly processed product, BPC-157 has been shown to work very effectively when taken orally.

This circles back to the gym world. Much of the accumulated experience with these peptides over the years has come from the gym-going and bodybuilding communities, and we owe them a debt of gratitude for helping pave the way to better understanding and usage. However, in the very early years of peptide use, they were only available in injectable forms. This history has created a persistent misconception that peptides must be injected to be effective. That is simply not true.

Longer peptides, such as those used for weight loss (like GLP-1 analogs), do require injection because they consist of much longer amino acid chains. But understand that the oral-formulation peptides discussed here work very well, are equally effective compared to injectable forms, and they are certainly more convenient. Consider the compliance factor: compliance rates are drastically better with oral peptides. After all, how likely is it that someone will consistently inject a peptide every morning and evening for months on end? Factor compliance into any comparison of efficacy.

Injectable peptides also raise concerns about sterility and proper handling. Additionally, injectable versions are typically available through research-only peptide suppliers (which aren't always trustworthy) or certain specialized pharmacies that are limited in what they can provide. Much of this regulation surrounding injectable peptides stems from concerns about sourcing them from research-only sites, where there have been reports of infections and adverse reactions from contaminated or improperly handled products.

All told, oral peptides are certainly much safer, more convenient, and promote better long-term compliance—all crucial factors for achieving optimal health outcomes.

And the field continues to evolve rapidly. I recently became aware of an oral weight loss peptide that should reach the market within the next year or two—an oral GLP-1 analog that appears to work equally well as the injectable versions. While it is currently only available for research purposes, this represents the broader trend toward effective oral peptide formulations.

The key takeaway is this: When you combine proper medical guidance, high-quality products, and the convenience of oral administration, peptides can be a remarkably safe and effective tool for optimizing your health and moving beyond merely treating disease to achieving optimal wellness.

At this point, I often hear another common question: How do I do this? How do I introduce peptides as a lifestyle?

Integrating Peptides into Daily Life

Making peptides part of the fabric of your day-to-day life—including a manageable and sustainable routine of meal prep, progress tracking, and positive mindset—can feel overwhelming. Fortunately, I'm happy to share a plan that, with the commitment to stick to it, you *can* use to achieve optimal health.

Here's how it works. First, remember that peptides aren't magic bullets that work in isolation. To truly optimize your health and see the dramatic improvements we've discussed throughout this book, you must first understand how peptides fit into the big picture of wellness. Think of peptides as the finishing touches on the dream home you've built—though incredibly powerful, they work best when applied to a solid foundation.

The Five Pillars of a Solid Foundation

Before we dive into peptide protocols, let's establish the foundational elements that will determine your success:

Diet forms the cornerstone of everything we are trying to accomplish. You can't supplement or peptide your way out of a poor diet. The foods you choose either fuel inflammation or fight it, support cellular repair or hinder it.

Sleep is when your body does its most important repair work. This is when many of the peptides we've discussed are naturally produced and when their signals are most effectively received by your cells.

Stress management—both spiritual and emotional—directly impacts your hormonal balance, immune function, and cellular communication. Chronic stress essentially creates static that interferes with the very signals peptides are designed to enhance.

Exercise provides the stimulus for adaptation and improvement. It's the trigger that tells your body it needs to get stronger, more resilient, and more efficient.

Strategic supplementation fills in the gaps where even excellent nutrition might fall short in our modern environment.

With those five pillars in place, you can incorporate supplements to help prioritize what matters most.

Adding Supplements

When it comes to supplements, I always start with the essentials before even considering peptides. Here's how I prioritize them:

Omega-3 fatty acids sit at the very top of this list. They are absolutely foundational for managing inflammation, supporting brain health, and optimizing cellular function. Without adequate omega-3s, many of the anti-inflammatory peptides we've discussed won't work as effectively. Phospholipids come right after omega-3s. These are crucial for cell membrane health and help ensure that the peptide signals can reach their target cells effectively. Curcumin from turmeric is another pretty important one. It works synergistically with many of the anti-inflammatory peptides, amplifying their effects while providing its own powerful benefits.

From there, I move into more individualized recommendations. For gut health—which impacts everything else—I typically recommend prebiotic vegetable fibers and probiotics, especially spore-based probiotics. These are very, very important for foundational health and optimizing overall wellness.

The key is having the right practitioner who can help customize what this supplement foundation looks like for your specific needs. But these basics give us a framework that helps you see everything clearly, prioritize what matters most, and ensure that important categories aren't missed.

Adding Peptides

Once the foundation is in place, we can develop a personalized plan for integrating peptides based on your specific needs. Keep in mind that this isn't a one-size-fits-all approach. Your peptide regimen should be as individual as your fingerprint, tailored to address your unique health challenges and optimization goals.

Part of that personalized plan depends entirely on what your blood work reveals and your specific health priorities. Are we focusing on gut healing? Immune optimization? Recovery enhancement? Each goal requires a different approach and different peptide combinations.

No matter the goal, they all demand one non-negotiable component: If you want to make lasting change, you need accountability. At the very least, be accountable to yourself through journaling. Do it every day, twice a week, even once a month. It might seem like a "chore" at first, but after you get in the habit, the simple act of transferring your thoughts to paper is wonderfully transformative and can be a powerful driver in making changes stick.

Yes, it's great to have data on your phone with fancy graphs and tracking apps, but there is something irreplaceable about sitting down and writing in a journal every day or two. It's a fine art that has been lost; many people don't recognize the full benefit anymore.

Consistency is Key

One thing I find myself emphasizing on a regular basis is a commitment to consistency on a daily basis. Here's an example from my practice:

Many of my patients have low melanocyte-stimulating hormone levels. The intervention there is the peptide KPV, and in most cases, I recommend they take it morning and evening until we recheck their level. I typically don't retest for four months, so I emphasize that, if they are going to do this, they commit to doing it consistently until we remeasure. Otherwise, it simply won't work.

When people follow through with that commitment, we see very consistent improvement. When they don't stick to the protocol, it's very hit and miss, and the majority don't see biomarker numbers change. This principle applies to every peptide protocol we implement. These compounds work through consistent signaling over time. Taking them sporadically is like having a conversation where you only say every third word—the message gets lost.

Throughout the entire process, tracking progress is another area of emphasis. It's not enough to just take peptides and hope for the best; you need concrete ways to measure improvement and adjust your approach accordingly.

In my practice, we schedule follow-up appointments three or four months later. That is when lab reports contrast previous results in one column and current results in another. It is always a powerful moment for patients to see this side-by-side comparison. I review the results with them, making notes and educating them about what we are seeing. They can easily observe the tangible progress they're making through blood tests that track their immune function, gut inflammation, melanocyte-stimulating hormone levels, and other key biomarkers.

This visual progress tracking serves multiple purposes. It validates that the protocols are working, provides motivation to continue, and gives us the data we need to fine-tune the approach going forward.

Putting It All Together

Remember, successful peptide integration isn't about adding one more pill to your routine. It's a comprehensive lifestyle approach where every element supports the other. Your diet supports your sleep, sleep enhances exercise recovery, stress management improves hormone balance and allows for healing, mitochondrial enhancement affects cellular efficiency throughout every system, and peptides amplify all these effects.

When patients approach it this way—with proper foundational support, consistent daily habits, accountability systems, and progress tracking—that's when we see the remarkable transformations peptides are capable of facilitating. This goes far beyond optimizing individual biomarkers to creating a sustained elevation in overall health and vitality that compounds over time.

Peptide integration goes far beyond optimizing individual biomarkers to creating sustained elevation in overall health and vitality.

The key is patience, consistency, and trust in the process. These changes don't happen overnight, but when you commit to the full approach, the results speak for themselves.

The Promise of Optimal Health: What You Can Expect

When people ask me what they can realistically expect from this comprehensive approach to health optimization, there's a long list of benefits they can anticipate. But let's start with the most immediate and noticeable change—a better sense of overall well-being.

Number one on that list is improved cognition—enhanced focus, faster processing speed, and clearer thinking. As I mentioned earlier in the book, the brain is incredibly metabolically active, so when we start reducing inflammation and improving mitochondrial function, we recognize it cognitively first. It's like removing a fog you didn't even realize was there. And this isn't a subtle change. We're talking about noticeable improvements in mental clarity, decision-making speed, and the ability to maintain focus throughout the day. Your brain literally has more energy to work with when inflammation decreases and cellular function improves.

Beyond the cognitive benefits, you can expect to see substantial physical improvements as well. If you have weight to lose or your metabolism has slowed, you can expect meaningful improvement in body composition. Particularly exciting in this area is when cravings begin to diminish significantly, from food cravings to more destructive hungers in the realm of addiction. Your energy levels will also improve dramatically, with sustainable, steady energy throughout the day rather than the peaks and crashes many people have grown accustomed to. Your skin will improve and develop that healthy glow that comes from optimal cellular function—visible signs of internal healing.

For the athletes out there, you can even measure improvements in VO2 max, which will likely increase as you optimize overall health, providing concrete data that your mitochondrial function and, subsequently, your cardiovascular system are functioning at a higher level.

Some of these improvements, and others, are noticed sooner than others. For example, someone with chronic conditions like eczema and asthma can expect those conditions to start improving within a four- to six-month timeframe. For others, it might take closer to a year to really optimize healing, but the trajectory is consistently upward when people commit to the process.

From a broader perspective, it's rare to find someone whose baseline health is already optimized. Most people, even those who consider themselves healthy, have significant room for improvement. As we improve health, reduce inflammation, optimize recovery, and do everything possible to enhance mitochondrial function, we can expect to see improvements in both strength and endurance that translate into real-world capabilities.

I experienced this in real time during a health challenge I faced earlier this year. I decided to pull out all the stops, committing to doing everything within my reach to get my health back. I implemented protocols from every angle we've discussed (and then some) to optimize my wellness, and the results exceeded my expectations. Recently, I went mountain biking near Park City with a good friend of mine. We're the same age; he's a family practice doctor as well, and for thirty years we've backcountry skied, biked, and hiked together all around Utah's high country. Typically, our fitness levels are very similar (at least before my illness knocked me down), but on this day, with perfect temps and ideal trail conditions, we huffed it over 3,000 vertical feet and then bombed down. Interestingly, I periodically had to wait for him on the way up, and at the top, it was a good ten minutes or so before he rejoined me. All told, at least on that day, I was quite a bit faster uphill than he was, and I attribute that to all the health optimization practices I was doing at the time (which was about everything imaginable). It not only brought me back to my previous baseline but raised it to a new level. I could really feel the improved strength and endurance that my rather extreme biohacking provided. Do I want to let off the gas? Do I want to eliminate any of my comprehensive regimen? Not just no, but "heck" no!

The takeaway goes far beyond personal metrics and performance improvements to a place where vibrant vitality is possible. This isn't about being selfish or self-focused (though I'll admit there were times in my life when my health optimization might have seemed that way). As we mature and have experiences that change our perspectives, we begin to see the big picture more clearly.

With genuine vitality—when your body and mind are functioning optimally—you can serve your community better, serve others more effectively, and progress in ways that seemed impossible before. You can offer so much more to society, to your family, to your friends, and ultimately to yourself.

Think about the last time you accomplished something meaningful when you had abundant energy versus running on empty. The difference is night and day. You offered something valuable and made something happen specifically because you had those vitality and energy reserves to draw upon.

What we are ultimately talking about here is creating a positive feedback loop. As your health improves, you have more energy to invest in the things that matter most to you. As you accomplish more meaningful work, you feel more purposeful and motivated to maintain these healthy practices. Serving others more effectively creates a sense of fulfillment that further supports your commitment to optimal health.

This is why I'm so passionate about this comprehensive approach. We aren't just trying to fix problems or treat symptoms. We are creating a foundation for you to become the fullest expression of who you are meant to be—physically, mentally, emotionally, spiritually, and in your contribution to the world around you.

•—•—•

Here's my challenge to you: Don't settle for "normal" health markers or "adequate" energy levels. Don't accept that declining vitality is just part of aging or that chronic inflammation is inevitable in our modern world. The tools we've discussed—proper nutrition, targeted supplementation, strategic peptide therapy, stress management, quality sleep, and consistent exercise—are not simply theoretical concepts. They are practical, proven interventions that can elevate your health to levels you might not have thought possible.

This approach works. You only need to commit to the process, trust in the timeline, and stay consistent with the practices that will get you there.

Your health is your power. Your life is your message. Live it well!

Acknowledgements

This book is the result of the collective wisdom, encouragement, and support of so many people, without whom it would never have been possible. I am deeply grateful to all who have contributed to its creation and to the ongoing journey of bringing *Big Picture Medicine* into practice.

To my godly parents (especially for my sweet mother, Noni)—thank you for instilling in me a passion for healing, for questioning the status quo, for deeply loving, serving, and guiding all within your reach. Thank you for your zest for life and for your quest to be optimally healthy and for enthusiastically sharing your knowledge with so many others. Thank you for guiding me toward a more integrative, functional approach to holistic healing.

To my mentors and teachers—I am indebted to the pioneers in functional medicine, chronic inflammatory response syndrome, peptide integration, and integrative wellness who have inspired me with their vision and courage. I will name some of you, knowing there are many more who have shaped my course: Mark Hyman, Dale Bredesen, Richie Shoemaker, Kent Holtorf, David Perlmutter, and Steven Gundry. Your insights continue to shape the way I think about health, resilience, and human potential.

To my patients and community—thank you for allowing me the privilege of walking alongside you on your journeys of healing. Your courage, perseverance, and trust have been my greatest teachers. This book exists because of the lessons you have shared and the hope you embody.

To my family and loved ones—words cannot fully express my gratitude. Thank you to my incredible wife, Kristin, for your unwavering patience, love, and encouragement, and to each of my children and grandchildren for reminding me of what truly matters. Your love and support sustained me through the long hours and hard work required to complete this project.

To the Ultimate Healer, Jesus Christ—most importantly, I have deep gratitude for my Savior, Jesus Christ. It is only through Him that we can be truly and completely healed, physically and spiritually. Through His mercy, His grace, and His resurrection, we can be transformed. I thank Our Father in Heaven for His consistent guidance and direction. Some call it "intuitive medicine," but I believe it to be Spirit-guided.

Finally, to everyone who believes that medicine can be more than symptom management—that it can be restorative, personalized, and transformative—this book is for you. May it serve as a resource and inspiration on the path toward optimal health and well-being.

About the Author

Stuart B. Porter, D.O. is a distinguished leader in functional medicine and regenerative therapies. He is board certified in family medicine and a fellow of the American Academy of Family Physicians. A graduate of Brigham Young University (B.S., Design Engineering, 1984) and Kirksville College of Osteopathic Medicine (D.O., 1988, graduating first in his class), Dr. Porter went on to complete his family medicine residency at Madigan Army Medical Center in 1993.

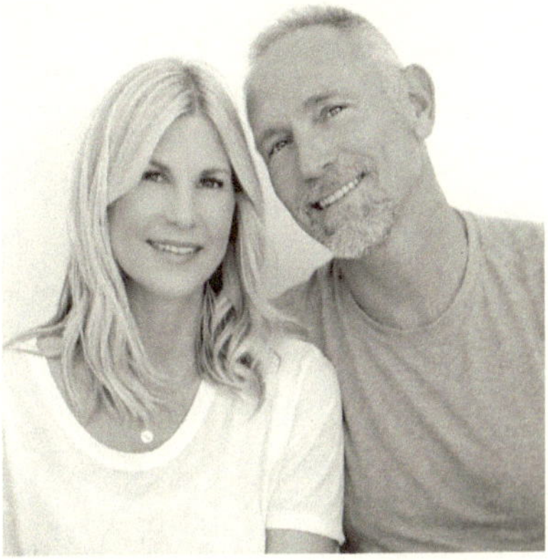

From 2003 to 2021, he served as regional dean for A.T. Still University's Kirksville College of Osteopathic Medicine in the Utah Region, mentoring hundreds of medical students over decades of academic leadership. He is certified in peptide therapy through the **Seeds Scientific Research & Performance (SSRP) Institute** and has become a trusted voice in integrating advanced peptide science with functional and regenerative medicine.

Dr. Porter is the founder of **Integrative Medical Associates** in Provo, Utah, and cofounder of **Xage Medical Spa**, a regenerative aesthetics practice. His clinical protocols have helped elite athletes, entertainers, and individuals from all walks of life achieve peak performance, longevity, and optimal health.

Beyond medicine, Dr. Porter is an accomplished endurance athlete. He has competed in numerous Ironman Triathlon races, qualifying for the Ironman World Championship five times. In 2017, he was ranked first in the United States and fourth in the world for full-distance Ironman competition. His passions include backcountry skiing, mountain biking, boating with family and friends, and embracing the outdoors as part of a lifelong commitment to fitness and vitality. He loves serving in his religious community and spending time with his wife of forty-three fabulous years, his five children, and nine (two of those are on their way!) grandchildren.

With *Big Picture Medicine: Optimizing Health and Wellness Through Functional Medicine and Peptide Integration*, Dr. Porter shares his clinical insights, athletic experience, and dedication to helping others unlock their full potential for health and well-being.

Notes

1 The George Washington Center for Integrative Medicine, "Shoemaker Protocol for Mold Toxicity and CIRS" accessed April 24, 2025, https://gwcim.com/services/shoemaker-protocol-cirs-mold-toxicity/.

2 Kent Holtorf, *Mold Illness and the Holtorf Updated Peptide Protocol for the Rapid Treatment of CIRS (HUPPRTOC)* (Holtorf Medical Group, 2023).

3 Naviaux RK. "Perspective: Cell Danger Response Biology—The New Science that Connects Environmental Health with Mitochondria and the RISING TIDE of Chronic Illness," *Mitochondrion* 51, (2020):40–45. doi: 10.1016/j.mito.2019.12.005. Epub 2019 Dec 23. PMID: 31877376.

4 Tracy Binius, "Treating Depression After a Heart Attack." *Northwestern Medicine*, April 2023. https://www.nm.org/healthbeat/healthy-tips/treating-depression-after-a-heart-attack.

5 Anna Jones, "How Giving to Others Can Boost Mental and Physical Health." *UAB News*, December 2, 2024. https://www.uab.edu/news/news-you-can-use/how-giving-to-others-can-boost-mental-and-physical-health.

6 Robert H. Shmerling, "Gratitude Enhances Health, Brings Happiness—and May Even Lengthen Lives." *Harvard Health Blog*, September 11, 2024. https://www.health.harvard.edu/blog/gratitude-enhances-health-brings-happiness-and-may-even-lengthen-lives-202409113071.

7 Chen Y, Okereke OI, Kim ES, Tiemeier H, Kubzansky LD, VanderWeele TJ, "Gratitude and Mortality Among Older US Female Nurses," *JAMA Psychiatry* 81, no. 10 (2024):1030–1038. doi:10.1001/jamapsychiatry.2024.1687

8 Karen Swartz, "Forgiveness: Your Health Depends on It." *Johns Hopkins Medicine*, last modified April 2024. https://www.hopkinsmedicine.org/health/wellness-and-prevention/forgiveness-your-health-depends-on-it.

9 Pew Research Center. 2019. *Religion's Relationship to Happiness, Civic Engagement and Health Around the World.* January 31. https://www.pewresearch.org/religion/2019/01/31/religions-relationship-to-happiness-civic-engagement-and-health-around-the-world/.

10 McLean Hospital, "Understanding Spirituality and Mental Health." Last modified October 18, 2024. https://www.mcleanhospital.org/essential/spirituality.

11 BiotiQuest, "History and Growth of Fermented Foods." Last modified June 2, 2025. https://biotiquest.com/blogs/blog/history-and-growth-of-fermented-foods.

12 HJ Wu, E Wu, "The Role of Gut Microbiota in Immune Homeostasis and Autoimmunity," *Gut Microbes* 3, no. 1 (2012):4–14. doi: 10.4161/gmic.19320. Epub 2012 Jan 1. PMID: 22356853; PMCID: PMC3337124.

13 Collet JP, Ducruet T, Floret D, Cogan-Collet J, Honneger D, Boissel JP, "Daycare Attendance and Risk of First Infectious Disease," *Eur J Pediatr* 150, no. 3 (1991):214–6. doi: 10.1007/BF01963570. PMID: 2044595.

14 Sambucol USA. "Mind-Body Connection and the Immune System." *Sambucol*, accessed June 12, 2025. https://sambucolusa.com/blogs/news/mind-body-connection-immune-system.

15 Nipunie S. Rajapakse and Jason H. Homme, *Ear Infections: If Not Antibiotics, Then What?* (Mayo Clinic Press), last modified August 2023. https://mcpress.mayoclinic.org/parenting/ear-infections-if-not-antibiotics-then-what//.

16 Healthline Editorial Team, n.d. "Does Exercise Boost the Immune System?" Healthline. Accessed June 14, 2025. https://www.healthline.com/nutrition/does-exercise-boost-immune-system.

17 Nieman DC, Wentz LM, "The Compelling Link Between Physical Activity and the Body's Defense System, *J Sport Health Sci* 8,no. 3 (2019):201–217. doi: 10.1016/j.jshs.2018.09.009. Epub 2018 Nov 16. PMID: 31193280; PMCID: PMC6523821.

18 Patti Neighmond, 2018. "How Much Protein Do You Really Need?" NPR, December 3, 2018. https://www.npr.org/sections/thesalt/2018/12/03/669808699/how-much-protein-do-you-really-need.

19 Weston A. Price. *Nutrition and Physical Degeneration*, 6th ed. (Price-Pottenger Nutrition Foundation, 2008).

20 Eric Suni, "How Sleep Affects Immunity." Sleep Foundation. Last modified August 15, 2023. Accessed June 15, 2025. https://www.sleepfoundation.org/physical-health/how-sleep-affects-immunity.

21 IMMUSE Health. "How Your Emotions Affect Your Body's Immune Response." Accessed June 15, 2025. https://immusehealth.com/news/post/how-your-emotions-affect-your-bodys-immune-response.

22 Debra Umberson and Jennifer Karas Montez, "Social Relationships and Health: A Flashpoint for Health Policy." Journal of Health and Social Behavior, 51, no. Suppl (2010): S54–66. https://doi.org/10.1177/0022146510383501.

23 RM Wilder. The effects of ketonemia on the course of epilepsy. Mayo Clinic Proceedings 6, (1921):307–308.

24 National Institute of Neurological Disorders and Stroke. "Brain Basics: Understanding Sleep." Accessed June 16, 2025. https://www.ninds.nih.gov/health-information/public-education/brain-basics/brain-basics-understanding-sleep.

25 Dale Bredesen, *The End of Alzheimer's Program: The First Protocol to Enhance Cognition and Reverse Decline at Any Age* (Avery, 2020).

26 Harvard Health Publishing, "Exercise Can Boost Your Memory and Thinking Skills." Harvard Health. Last modified August 26, 2024. https://www.health.harvard.edu/mind-and-mood/exercise-can-boost-your-memory-and-thinking-skills.

27 Chris Palmer, *Brain Energy: A Revolutionary Breakthrough in Understanding Mental Health--and Improving Treatment for Anxiety, Depression, OCD, PTSD, and More*, (BenBella Books, 2022).

28 Javadov, Sabzali, Andrey V. Kozlov, and Andreia S. Camara, "Mitochondria in Health and Diseases," *Cells* 9, no. 5 (2020): 1177. https://doi.org/10.3390/cells9051177.

29 Amy Myers, "Why It's Important to Maintain Mitochondrial Health." Amy Myers MD. October 14, 2024; Accessed June 26, 2025. https://www.amymyersmd.com/blogs/articles/mitochondrial-health.

30 Lucia Koklesova, Andrea Mazurakova, Marek Samec, Erika Kudela, Katarina Biringer, Peter Kubatka, and Olga Golubnitschaja, "Mitochondrial Health Quality Control: Measurements and Interpretation in the Framework of Predictive, Preventive, and Personalized Medicine," *EPMA Journal* 13, no. 2 (2022): 177–193. https://doi.org/10.1007/s13167-022-00281-6.

31 Javadov, Sabzali, Andrey V. Kozlov, and Andreia K. S. Camara, "Mitochondria in Health and Diseases," *Cells* 9, no. 5 (2020): 1177. https://doi.org/10.3390/cells9051177.

32 Allay Health & Wellness, "The Brain Energy Theory: A New Understanding of Mental Health." *Allay Health & Wellness*, February 18, 2025. Accessed June 26, 2025. https://allayhealthwellness.com/the-brain-energy-theory-a-new-understanding-of-mental-health/

33 Chris Palmer, *Brain Energy: A Revolutionary Breakthrough in Understanding Mental Health—and Improving Treatment for Anxiety, Depression, OCD, PTSD, and More* (BenBella Books, 2022).

34 Spectra Wellness, "Supplements & Therapies for Mitochondrial Support." *Spectra Wellness*, n.d. Accessed June 26, 2025. https://spectrawellness.com/supplements-therapies-for-mitochondrial-support/

35 Advisory Board, "Exercise vs. Antidepressants: Which Is Better at Treating Depression?" *Advisory Board Daily Briefing*, February 20, 2024. Accessed June 26, 2025. https://www.advisory.com/daily-briefing/2024/02/20/exercise-depression

36 Centers for Disease Control and Prevention, "Heart Disease Facts." October 2024. Accessed July 9, 2025. https://www.cdc.gov/heart-disease/data-research/facts-stats/index.html.

37 Centers for Disease Control and Prevention, "Stroke Facts." October 2024. Accessed July 9, 2025. https://www.cdc.gov/stroke/data-research/facts-stats/index.html.

38 Alzheimer's Disease International, "Dementia Statistics." Accessed July 9, 2025. https://www.alzint.org/about/dementia-facts-figures/dementia-statistics/.

39 R De Cabo and MP Mattson, "Effects of Intermittent Fasting on Health, Aging, and Disease," *New England Journal of Medicine* 381, no. 26 (2019):2541–2551

40 Danielle Masterson, NutraIngredients-USA. "Study Finds Most Americans Low in Omega-3 Fatty Acids, Could Impact Mood." May 24, 2021. https://www.nutraingredients-usa.com/Article/2021/05/24/Study-finds-most-Americans-low-in-omega-3-fatty-acids-could-impact-mood/.

MAISON VERO

Representing a community of authors whose books have collectively sold hundreds of millions of copies, the founders of The Gray + Miller Agency launched Maison Vero, a professional publishing house that partners with rising authors to bring their thought leadership to the world. Our representation covers every aspect of thought leadership, including U.S. senators, governors, and ambassadors, billionaire founders and entrepreneurs, researchers, academics, scientists, consultants, practitioners, social influencers, C-suite leaders, adventurers, professional athletes, artists, and creators. We partner with thought leaders and world changers like you who have a story to tell. By bringing decades of professional expertise to our clients, we are charting a new path in a timeless industry that transcends publishing norms, transforming powerful thoughts into impactful books that inspire minds, ignite hearts, and open doors.

Visit maisonvero.com to view our growing list of authors, or to submit a proposal for publication consideration.

Follow Maison Vero for insight and inspiration on social media:

MaisonVero MaisonVero MaisonVeroPublishing

For information about special discounts for bulk purchases, please call (949) 333-4872 or email info@graymilleragency.com.

Maison Vero is a partner brand of The Gray + Miller Agency, a speaking, literary, and talent consortium. For more information on the talent represented by The Gray + Miller Agency, or to bring any of our thought leaders to your organization or live event, please visit our website at **graymilleragency.com**.

www.ingramcontent.com/pod-product-compliance
Lightning Source LLC
LaVergne TN
LVHW091514200926
848483LV00008B/460/J
* 9 7 8 1 9 6 9 5 0 8 4 1 7 *